Toolbox for Autologous Breast Reconstruction

Guest Editor

MAURICE Y. NAHABEDIAN, MD

CLINICS IN PLASTIC SURGERY

www.plasticsurgery.theclinics.com

April 2011 • Volume 38 • Number 2

SAUNDERS an imprint of ELSEVIER, Inc.

W.B. SAUNDERS COMPANY
A Division of Elsevier Inc.

1600 John F. Kennedy Boulevard ● Suite 1800 ● Philadelphia, Pennsylvania 19103-2899

http://www.theclinics.com

CLINICS IN PLASTIC SURGERY Volume 38, Number 2
April 2011 ISSN 0094-1298, ISBN-13: 978-1-4557-0982-3

Editor: Joanne Husovski
Developmental Editor: Teia Stone

Clinics in Plastic Surgery (ISSN 0094-1298) is published quarterly by Elsevier Inc., 360 Park Avenue South, New York, NY 10010-1710. Months of issue are January, April, July, and October. Business and Editorial Offices: 1600 John F. Kennedy Blvd., Suite 1800, Philadelphia, PA 19103-2899. Periodicals postage paid at New York, NY and additional mailing offices. Subscription prices are $411.00 per year for US individuals, $617.00 per year for US institutions, $203.00 per year for US students and residents, $467.00 per year for Canadian individuals, $721.00 per year for Canadian institutions, $530.00 per year for international individuals, $721.00 per year for international institutions, and $256.00 per year for Canadian and foreign students/residents. To receive student/resident rate, orders must be accompanied by name of affiliated institution, date of term, and the *signature* of program/residency coordinator on institution letterhead. Orders will be billed at individual rate until proof of status is received. Foreign air speed delivery is included in all *Clinics* subscription prices. All prices are subject to change without notice. **POSTMASTER:** Send address changes to *Clinics in Plastic Surgery*, Elsevier Health Sciences Division, Subscription Customer Service, 3251 Riverport Lane, Maryland Heights, MO 63043. **Customer Service: 1-800-654-2452 (US and Canada). From outside of the United States and Canada, call 314-447-8871. Fax: 314-447-8029. E-mail: JournalsCustomerService-usa@elsevier.com (for print support); JournalsOnlineSupport-usa@elsevier.com (for online support).**

Reprints. For copies of 100 or more of articles in this publication, please contact the Commercial Reprints Department, Elsevier Inc., 360 Park Avenue South, New York, New York 10010-1710. Tel.: (+1) 212-633-3812; Fax: (+1) 212-462-1935; E-mail: reprints@elsevier.com.

Clinics in Plastic Surgery is covered in *Current Contents, EMBASE/Excerpta Medica, Science Citation Index, MEDLINE/ PubMed (Index Medicus), ASCA, and ISI/BIOMED.*

Printed and bound by CPI Group (UK) Ltd, Croydon, CR0 4YY

Transferred to Digital Print 2011

Contributors

GUEST EDITOR

MAURICE Y. NAHABEDIAN, MD, FACS
Associate Professor of Plastic Surgery,
Department of Plastic Surgery, Johns Hopkins
University, Georgetown University Hospital,
Washington, DC

AUTHORS

ROBERT J. ALLEN, MD
Department of Plastic Surgery, New York Eye
and Ear Infirmary; Center for Microsurgical
Breast Reconstruction, New York, New York

XAVIER ALOMAR, MD, PhD
Radiologist Consultant, Radiology Department,
Clínica Creu Blanca, Barcelona, Spain

MARK W. ASHTON, MBBS, MD, FRACS
The Taylor Laboratory, Jack Brockhoff
Reconstructive Plastic Surgery Research Unit,
Department of Anatomy and Cell Biology,
The University of Melbourne, Parkville,
Victoria, Australia

MAZEN I. BEDRI, MD
Plastic and Reconstructive Surgery at Mercy
Medical Center, Baltimore, Maryland

WILLIAM J. CASEY III, MD
Assistant Professor of Plastic and
Reconstructive Surgery, Division of Plastic and
Reconstructive Surgery, Mayo Clinic in
Arizona, Phoenix, Arizona

BERNARD W. CHANG, MD
Director, Plastic and Reconstructive Surgery at
Mercy Medical Center, Baltimore, Maryland

DANIEL CHUBB, MBBS (Hons), BMedSc
The Taylor Laboratory, Jack Brockhoff
Reconstructive Plastic Surgery Research Unit,
Department of Anatomy and Cell Biology,
The University of Melbourne, Parkville,
Victoria, Australia

JUAN A. CLAVERO, MD, PhD
Radiologist Consultant, Radiology
Department, Clínica Creu Blanca, Barcelona,
Spain

EMIL I. COHEN, MD
Division of Interventional Radiology,
Department of Radiology, Georgetown
University Hospital, Washington, DC

AMY S. COLWELL, MD
Assistant Professor, The Division of Plastic
Surgery, Harvard Medical School,
Massachusetts General Hospital, Boston,
Massachusetts

RANDALL O. CRAFT, MD
The Division of Plastic Surgery, Massachusetts
General Hospital, Boston, Massachusetts

LOUIS DE WEERD, MD, PhD
Plastic Surgeon, Department of Plastic Surgery
and Hand Surgery, University Hospital North
Norway, Tromsø, Norway

DAVID T. GREENSPUN, MD
Department of Plastic Surgery, New York
Eye and Ear Infirmary; Center for Microsurgical
Breast Reconstruction, New York, New York

DAMIEN GRINSELL, MBBS, FRACS
The Taylor Laboratory, Jack Brockhoff
Reconstructive Plastic Surgery Research Unit,
Department of Anatomy and Cell Biology,
The University of Melbourne, Parkville,
Victoria, Australia

GEOFFREY G. HALLOCK, MD
Division of Plastic Surgery, Sacred Heart
Hospital and The Lehigh Valley Hospitals,
Allentown; St. Luke's Hospital, Bethlehem,
Pennsylvania

ALEX KELLER, MD
Assistant Clinical Professor, Division of Plastic
Surgery, Department of Surgery, North Shore
Long Island Jewish Health System, New Hyde
Park; Division of Plastic Surgery, Department
of Surgery, New York University Medical
Center, New York, New York

PETER A. KREYMERMAN, MD
Instructor of Plastic and Reconstructive
Surgery, Division of Plastic and Reconstructive
Surgery, Mayo Clinic in Arizona, Phoenix,
Arizona

JUSTIN S. LEE, MD
Division of Vascular and Interventional
Radiology, Department of Radiology,
Georgetown University Hospital,
Washington, DC

JOSHUA L. LEVINE, MD
Department of Plastic Surgery, New York Eye
and Ear Infirmary; Center for Microsurgical
Breast Reconstruction, New York, New York

LUIS H. MACIAS, MD
Resident in Plastic and Reconstructive
Surgery, Division of Plastic and Reconstructive
Surgery, Mayo Clinic in Arizona, Phoenix,
Arizona

JAUME MASIA, MD, PhD
Professor and Chief, Plastic Surgery
Department, Hospital de la Santa Creu i Sant
Pau (Universidad Autónoma de Barcelona),
Barcelona, Spain

JAMES B. MERCER, PhD
Cardiovascular Research Group, Department
of Medical Biology, Faculty of Health Sciences,
University of Tromsø; Department of
Radiology, University Hospital North Norway,
Tromsø, Norway

MAURICE Y. NAHABEDIAN, MD, FACS
Associate Professor of Plastic Surgery,
Department of Plastic Surgery, Johns Hopkins
University, Georgetown University Hospital,
Washington, DC

CARMEN NAVARRO, MD
Plastic Surgery Consultant, Plastic Surgery
Department, Hospital de la Santa Creu i Sant
Pau (Universidad Autónoma de Barcelona),
Barcelona, Spain

TIFFANY M. NEWMAN, MD
Department of Radiology, Weill Cornell
Imaging, Weill Cornell and Columbia
University, New York, New York

KETAN M. PATEL, MD
Department of Plastic Surgery, Johns
Hopkins University, Georgetown University
Hospital, Washington, DC

MARTIN R. PRINCE, MD, PhD, FACR
Professor of Radiology, Weill Medical
College of Cornell University; Professor of
Radiology, Columbia College of Physicians
and Surgeons; Chief of MRI, New York
Hospital, New York, New York

ALANNA M. REBECCA, MD
Assistant Professor of Plastic and
Reconstructive Surgery, Division of
Plastic and Reconstructive Surgery,
Mayo Clinic in Arizona,
Phoenix, Arizona

**WARREN M. ROZEN, MBBS, BMedSc,
PGDipSurgAnat, PhD**
The Taylor Laboratory, Jack Brockhoff
Reconstructive Plastic Surgery
Research Unit, Department of
Anatomy and Cell Biology,
The University of Melbourne,
Parkville, Victoria, Australia

DAVID G. RUSCH, MD
Department of Radiology, Weill Cornell
Imaging at New York Presbyterian Hospital,
Weill Cornell and Columbia University,
New York; Department of Radiology,
White Plains Hospital, White Plains,
New York

MICHEL SAINT-CYR, MD, FRCS(C)
Associate Professor, Department of Plastic
Surgery, University of Texas Southwestern
Medical Center at Dallas, Dallas, Texas

JULIE V. VASILE, MD
Department of Plastic Surgery, New York Eye
and Ear Infirmary, New York, New York;
Department of Surgery, Stamford Hospital,
Stamford, Connecticut; Center for Microsurgical
Breast Reconstruction, New York, New York

SVEN WEUM, MD
Radiologist, Department of Radiology,
University Hospital North Norway;
Cardiovascular Research Group,
Department of Medical Biology, Faculty
of Health Sciences, University of Tromsø,
Tromsø, Norway

MICHAEL R. ZENN, MD, FACS
Vice Chief, Plastic and Reconstructive Surgery,
Duke University Medical Center, Durham,
North Carolina

ZHITONG ZOU, MD
Department of Radiology, Weill Cornell
Imaging at New York Presbyterian Hospital,
New York, New York

Contents

Minimizing Obstacles and Maximizing Outcomes in Microvascular Breast Reconstruction   xiii

Maurice Y. Nahabedian

Overview of Perforator Imaging and Flap Perfusion Technologies   165

Maurice Y. Nahabedian

Breast reconstruction has become an important consideration for women after mastectomy. Over the past decade, there have been a variety of technological advancements that have facilitated the ability to deliver reproducible and predictable outcomes with autologous breast reconstruction. This article chronicles many of the technological advancements and reviews the current toolbox that surgeons now have at their disposal when performing autologous reconstruction. It focuses on preoperative, intraoperative, and postoperative tools that have enabled the achievement of more reliable and predictable outcomes, especially in the setting of microvascular breast reconstruction.

Assessing Perforator Architecture   175

Michel Saint-Cyr

A myriad of options exist for autologous tissue perforator-based breast reconstruction. Each perforator selected has its distinct vascular territory, and proper knowledge of perforator perfusion characteristics helps maximize outcome and limit complications.

Acoustic Doppler Sonography, Color Duplex Ultrasound, and Laser Doppler Flowmetry as Tools for Successful Autologous Breast Reconstruction   203

Geoffrey G. Hallock

The sine qua non to best ensure viability of any autogenous tissues used for breast reconstruction is to maximize the appropriate circulatory pattern to that tissue. This overview of tools used in this regard, all based on the physical principles of the Doppler effect, compares the role today of acoustic Doppler sonography, color duplex ultrasound, and laser Doppler flowmetry for perforator identification and flap monitoring. The audible Doppler has recognized limitations, but remains the simplest and most universally available device to assist in this purpose. Laser Doppler flowmetry provides a reasonable system for both intraoperative and post-procedure objective monitoring of the chosen tissue transfer.

Maximizing the Use of the Handheld Doppler in Autologous Breast Reconstruction   213

Maurice Y. Nahabedian and Ketan M. Patel

The handheld acoustic Doppler is commonly used in the setting of autologous reconstruction. Like the color duplex Doppler, it can be used preoperatively but has the advantage of being used intraoperatively and postoperatively. It can be used as a sole modality or it can be used in conjunction with, or to confirm, the findings of CTA or MRA. This article focuses on the preoperative, intraoperative, and postoperative use of the handheld Doppler for free tissue transfer with an emphasis on perforator flap breast reconstruction.

Computerized Tomographic and Magnetic Resonance Angiography for Perforator-Based Free Flaps: Technical Considerations   219

Justin S. Lee, Ketan M. Patel, Zhitong Zou, Martin R. Prince, and Emil I. Cohen

Perforator-based free flaps rely on the appropriate dominant vessel supplying the vascular territory of the flap. Preoperative knowledge of the vascular anatomy can improve outcome and diminish surgical time. Several preoperative imaging techniques exist for surgical planning. Computed tomographic and magnetic resonance angiography are two emerging modalities that provide exceptional anatomic detail. Despite the growing utilization of cross-sectional imaging for preoperative planning, each modality has specific technical considerations that are necessary to consider in order to produce a quality study.

Computed Tomographic Angiography: Clinical Applications   229

Warren M. Rozen, Daniel Chubb, Damien Grinsell, and Mark W. Ashton

There has been a move towards increasingly refined techniques for autologous breast reconstruction, and given the substantial inter-individual variability of perforator anatomy, the need for reliable, accurate methods of vascular imaging has been sought. Computed tomographic angiography (CTA) can offer a range of applications in autologous breast reconstruction to aid surgical planning and improved outcomes. This article explores the utility of CTA in imaging perforators, pedicles and recipient vessels across a wide range of flap types and donor sites. CTA has a range of clinical applications in autologous breast reconstruction, and can aid operative planning and improve outcomes.

Computed Tomographic Angiography: Assessing Outcomes   241

William J. Casey III, Alanna M. Rebecca, Peter A. Kreymerman, and Luis H. Macias

Perforator flaps are preferable for breast reconstruction after mastectomy in many patients. Preoperative imaging of the perforators and source vessels is desirable to reduce surgeon stress, limit donor and recipient site complications, and minimize operative time and associated costs. Computed tomographic angiography (CTA) has been shown to provide highly accurate representations of vascular anatomy with excellent spatial resolution. A critical review of the currently available literature was performed to identify the benefits of preoperative imaging (specifically CTA) in perforator flap reconstruction.

Noncontrast Magnetic Resonance Imaging for Preoperative Perforator Mapping   253

Jaume Masia, Carmen Navarro, Juan A. Clavero, and Xavier Alomar

Identifying the position, course, and caliber of the dominant perforator is extremely valuable in the preoperative study for perforator surgery. Besides reliability, the ideal technique should offer low cost and high availability and reproducibility. It should be fast, easy to interpret, and free of morbidity. Multidetector-row computed tomography (MDTC) and magnetic resonance imaging (MRI) provide images that are easy to interpret, and assess the perforator's caliber and localization and its intramuscular course and anatomic relationships. Noncontrast MRI avoids radiation to the patient and eliminates the need for intravenous contrast medium. This article discusses this method and presents our experience.

Contrast-Enhanced Magnetic Resonance Angiography　　263

Julie V. Vasile, Tiffany M. Newman, Martin R. Prince, David G. Rusch,
David T. Greenspun, Robert J. Allen, and Joshua L. Levine

With technological advances in magnetic resonance angiography (MRA), spatial resolution of 1-mm perforating vessels can reliably be visualized and accurately located in reference to patients' anatomic landmarks without exposing patients to ionizing radiation or iodinated contrast, resulting in optimal perforator selection, improved flap design, and increased surgical efficiency. As their experience with MRA in breast reconstruction has increased, the authors have made changes to their MRA protocol that allow imaging of the vasculature in multiple donor sites (buttock, abdomen, and upper thigh) in one study. This article provides details of this experience with multiple donor site contrast-enhanced MRA.

Dynamic Infrared Thermography　　277

Louis de Weerd, James B. Mercer, and Sven Weum

This article describes how dynamic infrared thermography (DIRT) can be used in autologous breast reconstruction with a deep inferior epigastric perforator flap. This noninvasive and noncontact technique for indirect monitoring of skin blood perfusion can be used in the preoperative planning and intraoperative evaluation of flap perfusion, as well as the postoperative monitoring of perfusion dynamics of DIEP flaps. DIRT provides valuable information on the perfusion physiology of perforators.

Fluorescent Angiography　　293

Michael R. Zenn

Fluorescent angiography is a simple and effective real-time tool for measurement of tissue perfusion both in and out of the operating room. It has multiple uses including: (1) identifying perforating vessels during flap planning; (2) locating primary and secondary angiosomes within a prepared flap; (3) as an aid in decision making for tissue debridement and flap creation; (4) intraoperative evaluation of microanastomoses; (5) postoperative flap monitoring, and (6) documentation of perfusion. The technology is easy to use in the hands of the operating surgeon and is safe for the patient, as it requires no radiation exposure.

Near-Infrared Spectroscopy in Autologous Breast Reconstruction　　301

Amy S. Colwell and Randall O. Craft

Autologous breast reconstruction is commonly performed after mastectomy and provides a natural replacement that mimics the native breast. Although current free flap success rates exceed 95%, total flap loss can be devastating for patients. As a result, new technologies have emerged to provide an objective means for flap monitoring, with the hope that vaso-occlusive events can be detected before the clinical manifestation of a microvascular complication and the no-reflow phenomenon. This article focuses on the available data for one new technology, near-infrared spectroscopy, and its current use in clinical practice.

Use of the Implantable Doppler in Free Tissue Breast Reconstruction　　309

Mazen I. Bedri and Bernard W. Chang

In this article, the authors discuss the advances in monitoring free tissue transfers, with a focus on the implantable Doppler system. Authors address indications and techniques for implanting the Doppler system, in addition to presenting a framework to assess the reliability and potential benefits of the implantable Doppler device.

Noninvasive Tissue Oximetry   313

Alex Keller

Noninvasive tissue oximetry is playing an important role in postoperative monitoring of autologous tissue breast reconstruction flaps. It is increasingly being used intra-operatively to assist in perforator selection, tissue mapping, and assessment of mastectomy skin flap viability. This article reviews the use of tissue oximetry for intraoperative decision making, flap physiology, and postoperative monitoring, and also comments on common flap complications.

Index   325

Clinics in Plastic Surgery

FORTHCOMING ISSUES

**Cosmetic Medicine and Minimally
Invasive Surgery/State of the Art**
Malcolm D. Paul, MD, FACS,
Raffi Hovsepian, MD, and
Adam Rotunda, MD, *Guest Editors*

Functional Hand Reconstruction
Michael W. Neumeister, MD, FRCSC, FACS,
Guest Editor

RECENT ISSUES

January 2011

Vascular Anomalies
Arin K. Greene, MD, MMSc, and
Chad A. Perlyn, MD, PhD, *Guest Editors*

October 2010

Perforator Flaps
Peter C. Neligan, MB, BCh, FRCS(I), FRCS(C), FACS,
Guest Editor

July 2010

Abdominoplasty
Al Aly, MD, FACS, *Guest Editor*

THE CLINICS ARE AVAILABLE ONLINE!

Access your subscription at:
www.theclinics.com

Minimizing Obstacles and Maximizing Outcomes in Microvascular Breast Reconstruction

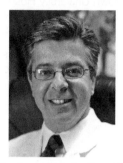

Maurice Y. Nahabedian, MD
Guest Editor

During the era of pedicle musculocutaneous flaps, plastic surgeons performed operations such as the latissimus dorsi and the TRAM with confidence and regularity. We have now entered the era of microvascular perforator flap reconstruction as patients and surgeons have recognized the benefits of muscle preservation. Microvascular perforator flaps such as the DIEP, SGAP, and TUG are arguably more complicated to perform and have the potential for morbidities that include total flap necrosis, partial flap necrosis, and fat necrosis. As such, the number of surgeons performing these procedures has remained less than those performing pedicle flap reconstruction. Reasons have included selecting appropriate patients for microvascular breast reconstruction, uncertainty regarding perforator caliber and location, determining perfusion quality within a flap, and the subjectivity of postoperative flap monitoring. In order to facilitate surgeon confidence and ability to perform these microvascular operations,

a number of technological advancements have generated selective tools that have enabled microvascular surgeons to perform these operations with confidence and regularity.

Surgeons now have the ability to optimize patient selection, select suitable perforators, assess flap perfusion, and monitor flaps with accuracy and reliability. These tools can be applied preoperatively, intraoperatively, and postoperatively.

Preoperatively, it is now possible to identify perforators and map their course using devices that include computerized tomographic angiography, magnetic resonance angiography, color duplex ultrasound, and dynamic infrared thermography. Intraoperatively, it is possible to assess flap perfusion and minimize the incidence of fat necrosis using fluorescent angiography.

Postoperatively, monitoring tools such as near-infrared spectroscopy and the hand-held acoustic Doppler permit reliable information. Having these tools in our toolbox has enabled more surgeons to perform these microvascular operations with

Clin Plastic Surg 38 (2011) xiii–xiv
doi:10.1016/j.cps.2011.04.001

confidence and with the end result of optimizing surgical outcomes.

This issue of *Clinics in Plastic Surgery* is organized to provide an update of the existing technological advancements and how they are used to improve outcomes. I am grateful to all of the contributors of the various topics. They are all experts in the field who have made significant contributions to the specialty and literature. The current toolbox for autologous reconstruction will hopefully provide useful information for the novice and experienced microsurgeon when planning, executing, and monitoring free tissue transfer operations.

Maurice Y. Nahabedian, MD
Department of Plastic Surgery
Johns Hopkins University
Georgetown University Hospital
3800 Reservoir Road NW
Washington, DC 20007, USA

E-mail address:
DrNahabedian@aol.com

Overview of Perforator Imaging and Flap Perfusion Technologies

Maurice Y. Nahabedian, MD

KEYWORDS

- Perforator flap • Magnetic resonance angiography
- Fluorescent angiography
- Computed tomographic angiography

PERFORATOR IMAGING AND FLAP TECHNOLOGY

Breast reconstruction has become an important consideration for women after mastectomy. The current American Society of Plastic Surgeons' (ASPS) procedural statistics reveal that approximately 25% of reconstructions are performed using autologous tissue and 75% are performed using prosthetic devices.[1] Although autologous breast reconstruction is less commonly performed than prosthetic-based reconstruction, there are many circumstances in which its use is preferred and indicated. The discrepancies between autologous and prosthetic reconstruction based on ASPS statistics are because of a variety of reasons. Arguments for prosthetic reconstruction include its ease relative to autologous reconstruction, patient factors that include shorter hospitalizations and less recovery time, as well as good to excellent aesthetic outcomes. Although, autologous reconstruction is considered by many surgeons as superior to prosthetic-based reconstruction in terms of overall aesthetics, some view it as too complicated, technically challenging, and more time consuming. Thus, the challenge has been to make autologous reconstruction more efficient, predictable, and reproducible.

From a historical perspective, autologous reconstruction has been limited by several factors, including selecting ideal patients, optimizing flap selection, length of surgery, and donor site morbidities. Donor site morbidities such as weakness, bulge, and hernia were occasionally observed after the use of traditional musculocutaneous flaps such as the pedicled transverse rectus abdominis musculocutaneous (TRAM).[2] As free tissue transfer methods of breast reconstruction became popular, donor site issues became less frequent; however, other obstacles such as anastomotic patency, postoperative monitoring, and ensuring flap survival became relevant.

The evolution of free tissue transfer and perforator flaps can be chronicled to a period in which patients became increasingly concerned about the mentioned donor site morbidities that were related to complete harvest of the donor site muscles. Perforator flap surgery was the perfect solution to this issue because the muscles were completely preserved. However, performing perforator flap surgery has demanded an entirely new skill set that includes identification and selection of suitable perforator vessels, dissection of intramuscular perforators, assessment of flap perfusion based on one or several perforators, and reliable postoperative monitoring. As patient demand for perforator flaps increased, surgeons began searching for technologies and tools that would make these operations more predictable and reproducible as well as enable them to perform these flap surgeries more consistently.

Over the past decade, there have been a variety of technological advancements that have facilitated the ability to deliver reproducible and predictable outcomes with autologous breast reconstruction. Preoperative advancements have enabled surgeons to identify suitable perforators

Department of Plastic Surgery, Johns Hopkins University, Georgetown University Hospital, 3800 Reservoir Road NW, Washington, DC 20007, USA
E-mail address: DrNahabedian@aol.com

Clin Plastic Surg 38 (2011) 165–174
doi:10.1016/j.cps.2011.03.005
0094-1298/11/$ – see front matter © 2011 Elsevier Inc. All rights reserved.

and to determine the patency of primary source vessels, namely the inferior epigastric and internal mammary vessels. Intraoperative advancements have enabled surgeons to assess anastomotic patency, vessel flow, and flap perfusion. Postoperative advancements have facilitated the ability of surgeons and nursing staff to monitor flaps based on tissue flow characteristics and discriminate between arterial and venous flow disturbances.

This article chronicles many of these advancements and reviews the current toolbox that surgeons now have at their disposal when performing autologous reconstruction. Some of the earlier tools include the acoustic Doppler ultrasonography and color duplex Doppler, whereas some of the newer tools include computed tomographic angiography (CTA), magnetic resonance angiography (MRA), dynamic infrared thermography (DIRT), fluorescent angiography and near-infrared spectroscopy (NIR). This article focuses on preoperative, intraoperative, and postoperative tools that have enabled the achievement of more reliable and predictable outcomes, especially in the setting of microvascular breast reconstruction.

HISTORICAL OVERVIEW

Over the past several centuries, surgeons and anatomists have been curious about soft tissue vascularity and cutaneous circulation.[3] A variety of methods have been described to better understand circulatory patterns. Early studies used vascular injection techniques that included India ink, colored wax, and latex. Other methods included tissue corrosion that used various metals, resins, or acids. With the introduction of radiography, the vascular anatomy could be better understood using radiopaque agents such as barium sulfate and lead oxide.

The importance of optimizing tissue perfusion increased when plastic surgeons began moving tissues from one part of the body to another. Flaps such as the latissimus dorsi and TRAM allowed for the reconstruction of many complex deformities. These flaps were based on an axial or source vessel that had many tributaries that traversed through the muscle and the adipocutaneous layer. Although the course of the axial artery and vein were generally constant and well known, the architecture of the microcirculation was variable and relatively unknown. Thus, the early era of flap transfer resulted in several morbidities that ranged from fat necrosis, partial flap necrosis, and in a few cases, total flap necrosis.[4] Many of these morbidities were the result of inadequate tissue perfusion at the distal aspects of the flap because of poor microcirculation. Intent on understanding these microcirculatory patterns

and reducing morbidities, surgeons partnered with industry to develop specific tools that would allow a better understanding and appreciation of the anatomy and perfusion.

The need and evolution of technology in the setting of flap reconstruction can be traced to the evolution of perforator flaps. Historically, musculocutaneous flaps resulted in fat necrosis in 5% to 10% of cases; however, with perforator flaps, this percentage increased.[5] This increase is because with perforator flaps, the entire adipocutaneous component of the flap is based on 1 or 2 perforating vessels rather than several. Factors such as the number of perforators, location of the perforators, and caliber of the perforators became important. In an early study evaluating outcomes after deep inferior epigastric perforator (DIEP) flap breast reconstruction, Kroll[6] demonstrated fat necrosis in 62% of flaps. However, with experience and a better understanding of the perforator anatomy and circulatory patterns, this number was significantly reduced.

Anatomic studies classified the various types of perforators into 5 groups,[7] including the single direct perforator as used for the superficial inferior epigastric artery (SIEA) flap and the 4 indirect perforators that include the subcutaneous, muscle, perimysial, and septal flaps. Although this classification was useful, it still did not provide sufficient preoperative information regarding the location and perfusion capabilities.

PREOPERATIVE ASSESSMENT FOR FLAP SURGERY

There are many questions that arise when considering the role of preoperative imaging before flap surgery, the most important of which is whether or not it is necessary for all patients and whether or not it improves outcomes. The answers to these questions are arguable, but there is no question that imaging will provide useful information. Advocates of preoperative imaging cite that the accurate identification of perforators facilitates preoperative decision making. Both the sensitivity and positive predictive value are 99.6%.[8] Given that harvesting perforator flaps is a complex operation with very little room for error, a preoperative knowledge of the location of dominant perforators lessens and shortens the learning curve associated with predictably and successfully mastering this operation. Skeptics of preoperative imaging state that preoperative knowledge of the perforators does not guarantee success and that performance and mastery of the technical exercise is necessary.

At present, several modalities are available for the preoperative assessment of perforators.[9–18]

These include duplex and color duplex ultrasonographies, CTA, MRA, and DIRT. Although, these modalities provide useful information, other factors such as scheduling, cost, and convenience may be relevant factors. In some cases, preoperative imaging is associated with radiation, whereas in others, the imaging tests may yield erroneous information because accuracy depends on the patient position and respiratory phase. The remaining sections of this article focus on what has been learned from these modalities.

Duplex and Color Duplex Ultrasonographies

Perhaps the first tool that surgeons used for preoperative mapping was Doppler ultrasonography. Although there are many clinical applications for the Doppler, plastic surgeons were interested in the Doppler to map out perforating vessels throughout the cutaneous territory of a flap.[9–11,19–22] There were several early studies using color Doppler that provided useful information related to the location, caliber, and flow patterns of the perforators in the planning of the TRAM flap.[9–11,19,20] Cluster analyses demonstrated that perforators were located throughout the anterior abdominal wall with most dominant perforators being situated around the periumbilical area.[9] Perforators exceeding 2.2 mm were far fewer but were identifiable in all 4 quadrants of the anterior abdominal wall.

There were other benefits of using Doppler assessment. Information such as flow, direction, and velocity was easily determined. In a study evaluating flap perfusion in TRAM, DIEP, and superior gluteal artery perforator (SGAP), it was determined that the highest blood flow and velocity was achieved in the TRAM flap followed by the DIEP and SGAP flaps.[20] Specific flow measurements in various vessels were obtained and included the deep inferior epigastric artery (DIEA) (10.45 mL/min), the superior gluteal artery (9.95 mL/min), and the internal mammary artery (37.66 mL/min). The imaging could differentiate between venous and arterial signals.[20] The perforator detection was found to be 96% effective. The principle limitation of the color duplex ultrasonography was that it could not provide 3-dimensional or architectural detail of the perforator system. Giunta[22] reported a relatively high number of false-positive results (46%) using the hand-held Doppler for localization of perforators. In a comparative study evaluating Doppler ultrasonography and CTA, Rozen and colleagues[23] found that CTA was superior to Doppler based on visualization of the DIEA, its branching pattern, and the perforators.

CTA

Computerized tomography may in some ways represent the gold standard for preoperative imaging.[12–15,24] This was the first of the highly accurate methods of perforator assessment. The benefits of CTA include precise anatomic localization of the perforators and the course of the perforator through the muscle. The technique of CTA is straightforward and involves the intravenous injection of a contrast medium. No oral contrast is necessary. Using multislice computerized tomography, axial and coronal images demonstrating the vascular architecture are obtained (**Fig. 1**).

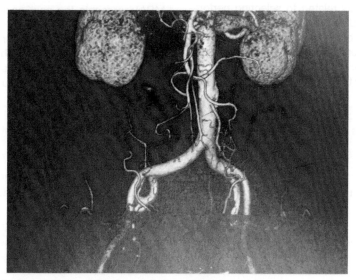

Fig. 1. CTA demonstrating patency of the deep inferior epigastric vessels.

This technique has proved reliable for preoperative assessment of the microcirculatory system and has provided valuable anatomic information as well.

The deep inferior epigastric vascular system has been well studied using the CTA. The traditional classification of the DIEA vessels included 3 types: type 1 occurred in 29% of patients and included a single vessel, type 2 occurred in 57% of patients and included a bifurcating vessel, and type 3 occurred in 14% of patients and included a trifurcating vessel.[25] This classification was modified based on the results obtained by using CTA in 498 abdominal walls. Rozen and colleagues[24] demonstrated that the DIEA branching pattern was different from that expected and developed a classification system based on 5 varieties. The groups included type 0 (<1%) in which the DIEA was absent, type 1 (43%) in which there was 1 DIEA trunk, type 2 (48%) in which there were 2 DIEA trunks, type 3 (9%) in which there were 3 DIEA trunks, and type 4 (<1%) in which there were 4 DIEA trunks. The relationship between the DIEA branching pattern and the perforators was also studied. Type 2 branching patterns were associated with a reduced transverse distance of the intramuscular portion of the perforator, whereas type 3 patterns exhibited an increased transverse distance.[24] The number of perforators was unrelated to the branching pattern.

There have been other clinical benefits related to the information generated using CTA. Casey[13] has demonstrated that preoperative CTA has had a beneficial effect on reducing the operative times and increasing the number of suitable perforators to be included in a flap and has reduced the incidence of a postoperative abdominal bulge. The latter is presumably related to selecting perforators in which the dissection would minimize injury to the innervation of the rectus abdominis muscle. Given that the intercostal innervation of the rectus abdominis muscle originates at the junction of the central and lateral thirds of the muscle, selection of medial rather than lateral perforators may reduce the incidence of nerve trauma. It was found that CTA had no beneficial effect on complications related to anastomosis, flap failure rates, occurrence of fat necrosis, and complications relayed to dehiscence or delayed healing.

CTA has been demonstrated to be a valuable tool in women who had prior abdominal surgery who are interested in DIEP flap reconstruction. Rozen and colleagues[26] studied 58 patients who had a total of 96 abdominal scars with CTA to determine if there was any disruption to the perforators or the primary source vessels. It was found that paramedian incisions invoked the most damage to the vascular supply, negatively affecting the perforators, SIEA, and DIEA vessels. On the contrary, laparoscopic incisions invoked the least damage. **Table 1** reviews the findings after CTA in the setting of different abdominal incisions.

The benefits of standard CTA are clearly evident. Advancements in computerized imaging have enabled the standard images to be reconstructed into a 3-dimmensional image.[15,27,28] The benefits of 3-dimensional imaging are that it permits accurate visualization of the right and left sides and may be useful when deciding between the right and left flap. It also provides information on whether to select medial or lateral row perforators. The correlation of 3-dimmensional imaging parallels the intraoperative anatomy and findings more accurately than standard CTA imaging. Finally, it may provide information that dissuades one from performing a perforator flap and choose instead to perform a muscle-sparing free TRAM.

MRA

MRA represents the next generation in vascular imaging.[16,17,29,30] This is in part because the imaging quality is maintained or enhanced without the aid of ionizing radiation. When compared with CTA, MRA has lower spatial resolution but greater contrast resolution.[29] This feature enables MRA to

Table 1
Effect of various abdominal incisions on the patency of the DIEA, SIEA, and perforating vessels

Scar	n	SIEA Disruption	DIEA Disruption	Perforator Disruption
Laparoscopy	20	None	None	None
Open Appendectomy	20	All (ipsilateral)	None (ipsilateral)	Medial row of DIEA
Pfannenstiel	35	Medial branch (30/35)	None	NR
Paramedian	3	All (ipsilateral)	All (ipsilateral)	All (ipsilateral)
Open Cholecystectomy	1	None	None	None
Midline	17	None	None	Crossover

Abbreviation: NR, not reported.

detect very small perforators that might otherwise not be visualized on CTA. Basically, MRA-produced images require magnetic fields, radio waves, and computers. High-quality images can be obtained with or without contrast agents. The benefit of MRA is that the quality of the vascular conduits or perforators as well as the flow patterns can be seen. This visualization is especially useful for perforator flaps virtually anywhere in the body. The main limitation of MRA is that motion can affect visualization. Patients must hold their breath during the imaging phase.

MRA enables the surgeon to become aware of the perforator location, size, and distance from the umbilicus. Chernyak and colleagues[29] described the utility of MRA in 21 patients undergoing DIEP flap reconstruction. Of these patients, 11 had bilateral DIEP flaps; therefore, 30 flaps were harvested. Axial, 3-dimensional, gadolinium-enhanced, T1-weighted, fat-suppressed, gradient-echo magnetic resonance images were obtained in all patients. Within the group of 21 patients, a total of 118 perforators were visualized with a mean diameter of 1.1 mm (range, 0.8–1.6 mm). Of these perforators, 30 were considered ideal. The mean diameter in this subgroup was 1.4 mm (range, 1–1.6 mm). These imaged perforators were then compared with operative findings. Intraoperatively, a total of 122 perforators were identified. All the 118 perforators seen on MRA were visualized. The 30 flaps were raised on 33 perforators that included a single-perforator flap in 27 and a double-perforator flap in 3. Of the 33 perforators that were harvested, 28 were considered ideal based on the preoperative MRA. Thus, there is good to excellent correlation (97%) between MRA and operative findings.

Other studies demonstrating the benefits of MRA for perforator flaps have been reported. Greenspun and colleagues[17] reviewed the outcomes in 31 women (50 flaps) scheduled for DIEP flaps. All perforators visualized on MRA using a gadolinium-based contrast agent were found intraoperatively. The specific intraoperative location of the perforators was within 1 cm of that predicted using MRA in 100% of patients. In 3 flaps, the DIEA perforators were small and the SIEA system was relatively large. MRA successfully predicted the preferred use of an SIEA flap instead of the DIEP flap in 3 of 3 women (100%). In the same study, the surgeons used a surface Doppler and found signals that corresponded to MRA findings in 44 of the 50 flaps. In 6 flaps, no Doppler signal was found preoperatively; however, intraoperatively, the perforator was clearly visualized in all 6 flaps.

Vasile and colleagues[30] demonstrated that a similar technology could be applied to the gluteal and upper thigh regions to determine the location of perforating vessels. They used a 1.5-T scanner rather than the 3.0-T scanner to improve image quality. MRA was used in 32 buttocks and imaged 142 perforators. The superior gluteal artery was the source for 92 (57.5%) perforators, the inferior gluteal artery for 56 perforators (35%), and the deep femoral artery for 11 (7.5%) perforators. The investigators concluded that MRA contributes to improved flap design based on the location and course of the perforating vessels. This information may determine whether an inferior or a superior gluteal perforator flap should be used.

Masia and colleagues[16] have used MRA without contrast agents and have obtained remarkably clear images of abdominal perforators. In 56 women having DIEP flap breast reconstruction, a dominant perforator was identified using MRA and correlated with intraoperative findings in all (100%). Using a refined imaging system, the investigators were able to accurately determine the location of the dominant perforator, define its intramuscular course, and reliably evaluate the SIEA and determine its dominance or lack thereof. The dominant perforator was paraseptal in 14% of flaps and intramuscular in 86% of flaps. Of the intramuscular perforators, the origin was from the lateral row in 55% and from the medial row in 31%.

DIRT

The concept of thermal imaging to assess cutaneous circulation is not novel. It has been used since the 1980s.[31,32] However, the application of thermal imaging to map out perforating vessels for the preoperative planning of DIEP flaps is novel. DIRT has been described and used for musculocutaneous and fasciocutaneous flaps but has only recently been used for the planning and mapping of perforator flaps.[18,33–35]

The technique of DIRT is straightforward. The principle is based on surface cooling (cold challenge) followed by a period of rewarming. This cold challenge causes relative hypoperfusion of the cutaneous surface. After termination of the cold challenge, the tissues naturally rewarm. As the tissues rewarm, an infrared camera analyzes the changes in cutaneous perfusion and localizes hot spots that correlate with the location of the perforating vessels. These hot spots are validated based on Doppler ultrasonography to ensure accuracy.

In the only clinical study to date evaluating the role of DIRT for preoperative planning, de Weerd and colleagues[18] evaluated 23 patients before having DIEP flap breast reconstruction. They found that it was the rate of rewarming that was critical to perforator selection. Perforators associated with rapid rewarming were more reliable than those associated with slow rewarming. They also concluded that the pattern of rewarming was important. Rapid rewarming associated with a progressive enlargement in the area was associated with the more dominant perforators. Other findings included a large number of perforators located at the tendinous inscriptions as well as in the lateral row. Of the 23 flaps, all were based on lateral row perforators, 14 were at the tendinous inscription, 9 were based on a single perforator, and 14 were based on 2 perforators. **Table 2** provides a comparison of the various preoperative imaging modalities.

INTRAOPERATIVE ASSESSMENT

Preoperative mapping of the perforators represents the first step in the performance of perforator flaps. The next logical step is to assess the perfusion of these flaps based on the primary blood supply. Traditionally, flap perfusion has been assessed by observing the color of the flap and determining the rate of capillary refill in the center and at the periphery of the flap. Other methods have included assessment of bleeding along the cut edges of the flap, which typically includes arterial and venous bleeding in equal proportions. Excessively dark venous blood with minimal or no arterial bleeding is a sign of poor perfusion. The main limitation with these methods of analysis is that there has not been a way to quantitate relative perfusion along the entire surface of the flap.

Fluorescent Angiography

Fluorescent angiography is a relatively new technology that allows for direct visualization of perfusion within a cutaneous territory.[36-43] This technique can be used on tissue that is elevated as a flap or on a cutaneous territory that has not been elevated. The images are captured after the intravenous injection of indocyanine green (ICG).

An image-capturing device is then positioned a few inches above the cutaneous territory to be imaged. This device is linked to a computer that analyzes the data and generates the real-time image. Images are obtained about 15 seconds after the ICG injection. In the setting of flap reconstruction, the images can be captured before flap elevation, during flap elevation, after flap elevation, and postoperatively. Fluorescent angiography has also been useful to assess the perfusion and viability of the mastectomy skin flaps as a means of minimizing skin necrosis.

One of the first applications of fluorescent angiography in the setting of autologous reconstruction was to confirm and validate the early studies that described the 4 zones of the TRAM flap. The original zones of the TRAM flap were reported by Scheflan and colleagues[44,45] and Hartrampf and colleagues[46] who described the 4 zones of an abdominal flap based on the presumed vascular perfusion. Zone 1 was based directly over the muscle or source vessel, zone 3 was adjacent and lateral to zone 1, zone 2 was just across the midline, and zone 4 was lateral to zone 3. Holm and colleagues[43] have revisited this traditional paradigm using video angiography and ICG. They demonstrated that abdominal flap zone based on this technique was different than previously thought. Zone 2 was actually lateral to zone 1 and zone 4 was lateral to zone 3.

Other clinical applications have included assessing the perfusion in various free tissue transfer operations. Pestana and colleagues[42] used fluorescent angiography in 23 patients with defects of the head and neck, breast, and extremities. Flaps included the TRAM, DIEP, SIEA, SGAP, lateral arm, anterolateral thigh, and latissimus dorsi. The safety and efficacy of the technique was demonstrated. The ability to assess perfusion at the distalmost aspects of muscle and musculocutaneous flaps was confirmed. Areas of the flap with relative hypoperfusion went on to develop small areas of necrosis or eschar formation. The

Table 2
Comparison of the various tools for assessing the characteristics of the source and perforating vessels

Test	Radiation Exposure	Contrast	Caliber	Location	Flow	Course	Accuracy
Doppler	No	No	No	Yes	No	No	Low
Color Duplex	No	No	No	Yes	Yes	No	Moderate
MDCTA	Yes	Yes	Yes	Yes	No	Yes	High
MRA	No	Yes	Yes	Yes	No	Yes	High
DIRT	No	No	No	Yes	Yes	No	Moderate

Abbreviation: MDCTA, multidetector computed tomographic angiography.

patency of the microvascular anastomosis was confirmed based on arterial inflow and venous outflow.

An almost equally important application of successful breast reconstruction using autologous reconstruction is predicting the viability of the mastectomy skin flaps. Predicting the viability of these skin flaps has always been challenging and when compromised could result in dramatic complications related to skin necrosis. In a recent article, the incidence of minor or major necrosis of the mastectomy skin flaps was 18.3%.[47] Komorowska-Timek and Gurtner[36] have evaluated the mastectomy skin flaps using fluorescent angiography. They found the technique to be beneficial, especially in cases of mastectomy with nipple-areolar preservation. Alterations in perfusion were noted in some women despite what appeared to be a normal nipple-areolar complex. All cases of poor perfusion based on fluorescent angiography, which were not debrided initially, went on to develop mastectomy skin flap necrosis in the corresponding areas. Jones and colleagues[38,40] have demonstrated that patients with a history of tobacco use or connective tissue disorders are more likely to have perfusion alterations of the skin flaps after mastectomy. These alterations can be predicted using fluorescent angiography.

POSTOPERATIVE ASSESSMENT

Postoperative assessment of flap circulation has traditionally required subjective interpretation of objective data. Traditional methods of flap monitoring have included hand-held Doppler probes, surface temperature assessment, flap turgor, capillary refill, and flap color.[48] Although these methods can be effective, they are usually not continuous, subject to interpretation, and depend on clinical personnel. It is also important to differentiate between arterial inflow and venous outflow problems. With inflow problems, the flap becomes pale, cool, and soft with delayed or absent capillary refill. With venous outflow problems, the flap becomes tense, congested, and purple, with brisk capillary refill. The reality of flap monitoring is that there is a short window of opportunity in which the flap can be salvaged in the event of altered flow. With a musculocutaneous or muscle flap, this window is typically about 2 hours. After 2 hours, there may be irreversible ischemic damage to muscle fibers, resulting is flap necrosis. With a perforator flap, this window of opportunity is increased and ranges from 3 to 6 hours because there is no muscle. The metabolic activity of skin and fat is less than that of muscle; therefore, these tissues are better able to tolerate ischemia.

NIR

NIR for monitoring free flaps has received considerable attention over the past several years.[49–51] This technology permits continuous monitoring of oxygen saturation within the cutaneous layer of the flap. A flat surface probe is placed on the skin, which emits near-infrared light (**Fig. 2**). This probe is able to detect the hemoglobin content in the surface vessels. This light has a maximum penetration depth of 2 cm. The probe is linked to a computer that translates the data into a linear measurement (**Fig. 3**). This measurement is constant for a given flap. Alteration in flow, including arterial or venous, is detected immediately, even before there are any clinical signs of altered flap perfusion.

Clinical application of this technology has been encouraging. Keller[50] has used NIR in 145 patients and 208 flaps. All patients were monitored intraoperatively and for 36 hours postoperatively.[50] Of the 208 flaps, 5 demonstrated abnormalities in the spectroscopy measurements. All these flaps were salvaged, in part because of the early diagnosis of altered perfusion. Colwell and colleages[49] applied NIR in 7 patients having free flap breast reconstruction using abdominal flaps. The baseline oxygen tension measurements ranged from 70% to 99% with a mean of 83%. Zone 1 readings remained unchanged after flap elevation; however, zone 4 readings were reduced by 15% to 20% (the mean oxygen tension being 64%). With clamping of the vessels to occlude flow, the measurements dropped by 25% to 38%. Saint-Cyr[52] has used NIR on mastectomy skin flaps. It was demonstrated that factors predisposing to skin necrosis included aggressive medial and inferior parenchymal resections as well as the length of the mastectomy flaps.

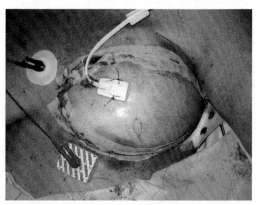

Fig. 2. Monitoring probe on the surface of a flap to detect changes in tissue oxygenation.

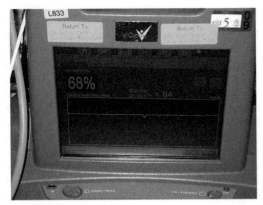

Fig. 3. The visual tracing of tissue oxygenation as achieved using NIR.

SUMMARY

The influx of technology has facilitated the ability to perform reconstructive procedures using autologous tissue. These technologies can be applied preoperatively, intraoperatively, and postoperatively. The reproducibility of these techniques has proved to be reliable and should increase the numbers of autologous reconstructions performed. The degree of accuracy in predicting the location and course of these perforators is unmatched based on conventional modalities. The quality of the images and the ability to easily translate this preoperative knowledge to the operating room is invaluable. Surgeons can now determine how much of a flap will survive based on intraoperative perfusion studies, which should reduce the incidence of fat necrosis. Using advancements in postoperative flap monitoring, surgeons and nurses can detect changes in tissue oxygenation and flow patterns earlier than they can using conventional methods. All these advancements have furthered the ability to perform reconstruction using microvascular techniques and are hoped to translate into improved outcomes.

REFERENCES

1. Plastic surgery procedural statistics. Available at: www.plasticsurgery.org. Accessed October 4, 2010.
2. Nahabedian MY, Manson PN. Contour abnormalities of the abdomen after transverse rectus abdominis muscle flap breast reconstruction: a multifactorial analysis. Plast Reconstr Surg 2002;109:81.
3. Bergeron L, Tang M, Morris SF. A review of vascular injection techniques for the study of perforator flaps. Plast Reconstr Surg 2006;117:2050.
4. Kroll SS, Gherardini G, Martin JE, et al. Fat necrosis in free and pedicled TRAM flaps. Plast Reconstr Surg 1998;102:1502–7.
5. Nahabedian MY, Tsangaris T, Momen B. Breast reconstruction with the DIEP flap or the muscle-sparing (MS-2) free TRAM flap: is there a difference? Plast Reconstr Surg 2005;115:436.
6. Kroll SS. Fat necrosis in free transverse rectus abdominis myocutaneous and deep inferior epigastric perforator flaps. Plast Reconstr Surg 2000;106:576.
7. Blondeel PN, Van Landuyt KH, Monstrey SJ, et al. The "Gent" consensus on perforator flap terminology: preliminary definitions. Plast Reconstr Surg 2003;112:1378.
8. Rozen WM, Ashton MW, Stella DL, et al. The accuracy of computed tomographic angiography for mapping the perforators of the DIEA: a cadaveric study. Plast Reconstr Surg 2008;122:363.
9. Chang BW, Luethke R, Berg WA, et al. Two-dimensional color Doppler imaging for precision preoperative mapping and size determination of TRAM flap perforators. Plast Reconstr Surg 1994;93:197.
10. Rand RP, Cramer MM, Strandness DE. Color-flow duplex scanning in the preoperative assessment of TRAM flap perforators: a report of 32 consecutive patients. Plast Reconstr Surg 1994;93:453.
11. Blondeel PN, Beyens G, Verhaeghe R, et al. Doppler flowmetry in the planning of perforator flaps. Br J Plast Surg 1998;51:202.
12. Alonso-Burgos A, García-Tutor E, Bastarrika G, et al. Preoperative planning of deep inferior epigastric artery perforator flap reconstruction with multislice-CT angiography: imaging findings and initial experience. J Plast Reconstr Aesthet Surg 2006;59:585–93.
13. Casey WJ, Chew RT, Rebecca AM, et al. Advantages of preoperative computed tomography in deep inferior epigastric artery perforator flap breast reconstruction. Plast Reconstr Surg 2009;123:1148.
14. Rozen WM, Palmer KP, Suami H, et al. The DIEA branching pattern and its relationship to perforators: the importance of preoperative computed tomographic angiography for DIEA perforator flaps. Plast Reconstr Surg 2008;121:367.
15. Masia J, Clavero JA, Larrañaga JR, et al. Multidetector-row computed tomography in the planning of abdominal perforator flaps. J Plast Reconstr Aesthet Surg 2006;59:594–9.
16. Masia J, Kosutic D, Cervelli D, et al. In search of the ideal method in perforator mapping: noncontrast magnetic resonance imaging. J Reconstr Microsurg 2010;26(1):29–35.
17. Greenspun D, Vasile J, Levine JL, et al. Anatomic imaging of abdominal perforator flaps without ionizing radiation: seeing is believing with magnetic resonance imaging angiography. J Reconstr Microsurg 2010;26(1):37–44.

18. de Weerd L, Weum S, Mercer JB. The value of dynamic infrared thermography (DIRT) in perforator selection and planning of free DIEP flaps. Ann Plast Surg 2009;63:274–9.

19. Berg WA, Chang BW, DeJong MR, et al. Color Doppler flow mapping of abdominal wall perforating arteries for transverse rectus abdominis myocutaneous flap in breast reconstruction: method and preliminary results. Radiology 1994;192:447.

20. Heitland AS, Markowicz M, Koellensperger E, et al. Duplex ultrasound imaging in free transverse rectus abdominis muscle, deep inferior epigastric artery perforator, and superior gluteal artery perforator flaps early and long-term comparison of perfusion changes in free flaps following breast reconstruction. Ann Plast Surg 2005;55:117–21.

21. Heller L, Levin S, Klitzman B. Laser Doppler flowmeter monitoring of free-tissue transfers: blood flow in normal and complicated cases. Plast Reconstr Surg 2001;107:1739.

22. Giunta RE, Geisweid A, Feller AM. The value of preoperative Doppler sonography for planning free perforator flaps. Plast Reconstr Surg 2000;105:2381–6.

23. Rozen WM, Phillips TJ, Ashton MW, et al. Preoperative imaging of DIEA perforator flaps: a comparative study of computed tomographic angiography and Doppler ultrasound. Plast Reconstr Surg 2008;121:1–8.

24. Rozen WM, Ashton MW, Grinsell D. The branching pattern of the deep inferior epigastric artery revisited in-vivo: a new classification based on CT angiography. Clin Anat 2010;23:87–92.

25. Moon HK, Taylor GI. The vascular anatomy of rectus abdominis musculocutaneous flaps based on the deep superior epigastric system. Plast Reconstr Surg 1988;82:815–32.

26. Rozen WM, Garcia-Tutor E, Alonso-Burgos A, et al. The effect of anterior abdominal wall scars on the vascular anatomy of the abdominal wall: a cadaveric and clinical study with clinical implications. Clin Anat 2009;22:815–23.

27. Pacifico MD, See MS, Cavale N, et al. Preoperative planning for DIEP breast reconstruction: early experience of the use of computerized tomography angiography with VoNavix 3D software for perforator navigation. J Plast Reconstr Aesthet Surg 2009;62:1464–9.

28. Gacto-Sánchez P, Sicilia-Castro D, Gómez-Cía T, et al. Computed tomographic angiography with VirSSPA three-dimensional software for perforator navigation improves perioperative outcomes in DIEP flap breast reconstruction. Plast Reconstr Surg 2010;125:24.

29. Chernyak V, Rozenblit AM, Greenspun DT, et al. Breast reconstruction with deep inferior epigastric artery perforator flap: 3.0-T gadolinium enhanced MR imaging for preoperative localization of abdominal wall perforators. Radiology 2009;250(2):414–24.

30. Vasile JV, Newman T, Rusch DG, et al. Anatomic imaging of gluteal perforator flaps without ionizing radiation: seeing is believing with magnetic resonance angiography. J Reconstr Microsurg 2010;26(1):45–57.

31. Theuvenet WJ, Koeyers GF, Borghouts MH. Thermographic assessment of perforating arteries. Scand J Plast Reconstr Surg 1986;20:25–9.

32. Wilson SB, Spence VA. Dynamic thermography imaging method for quantifying dermal perfusion: potential and limitations. Med Biol Eng Comput 1989;27:496–501.

33. Zetterman E, Salmi A, Suominen S, et al. Effect of cooling and warming on thermographic imaging of the perforating vessels of the abdomen. Eur J Plast Surg 1999;22:58–61.

34. Salmi A, Tukiainen E, Asko-Seljavaara S. Thermographic mapping of perforators and skin blood flow in the free transverse rectus abdominis musculocutaneous flap. Ann Plast Surg 1995;35:159–64.

35. Itoh Y, Arai K. Use of recovery-enhanced thermography to localize cutaneous perforators. Ann Plast Surg 1995;34:507–11.

36. Komorowska-Timek E, Gurtner GC. Intraoperative perfusion mapping with laser-assisted indocyanine green imaging can predict and prevent complications in immediate breast reconstruction. Plast Reconstr Surg 2010;125:1065.

37. Francisco BS, Kerr-Valentic MA, Agrawal JP. Laser-assisted indocyanine green angiography and DIEP breast reconstruction. Plast Reconstr Surg 2010;125(3):116e.

38. Jones GE. Laser-assisted indocyanine green angiography and DIEP breast reconstruction. In: Jones GE, editor. Bostwick: plastic and reconstructive breast surgery. St Louis (MO): QMP publishers; 2010. p. 1–15.

39. Murray JD, Jones GE, Elwood ET, et al. Fluorescent intraoperative tissue angiography with indocyanine green: the evaluation of nipple-areolar vascularity during breast reduction surgery [abstract]. Plast Reconstr Surg 2009;(Suppl 60):60.

40. Jones GE, Garcia CA, Murray J, et al. Fluorescent intraoperative tissue angiography for the evaluation of the viability of pedicled TRAM flaps. Plastic Reconstr Surg 2009;124(4):53.

41. Newman MI, Samson MC. The application of laser-assisted indocyanine green fluorescent dye angiography in microsurgical breast reconstruction. J Reconstr Microsurg 2009;25:21.

42. Pestana IA, Coan B, Erdmann D, et al. Early experience with fluorescent angiography in free-tissue transfer reconstruction. Plast Reconstr Surg 2009;123:1239.

43. Holm C, Mayr M, Höfter E, et al. Perfusion zones of the DIEP flap revisited: a clinical study. Plast Reconstr Surg 2006;117:37.

44. Scheflan M, Dinner MI. The transverse abdominal island flap: part I. Indications, contraindications, results, and complications. Ann Plast Surg 1983;10:24.

45. Scheflan M, Dinner MI. The transverse abdominal island flap: part II. Surgical technique. Ann Plast Surg 1983;10:120.

46. Hartrampf CR, Scheflan M, Black PW. Breast reconstruction with a transverse abdominal island flap. Plast Reconstr Surg 1982;69:216.

47. Chun YS, Verma K, Rosen H, et al. Implant-based breast reconstruction using acellular dermal matrix and the risk of postoperative complications. Plast Reconstr Surg 2010;125:429.

48. Smit JM, Zeebregts CJ, Acosta R, et al. Advancements in free flap monitoring in the last decade: a critical review. Plast Reconstr Surg 2010;125:177.

49. Colwell AS, Wright L, Karanas Y. Near-infrared spectroscopy measures tissue oxygenation in free flaps for breast reconstruction. Plast Reconstr Surg 2008;121:344e.

50. Keller A. A new diagnostic algorithm for early prediction of vascular compromise in 208 microsurgical flaps using tissue oxygen saturation measurements. Ann Plast Surg 2009;62:538–43.

51. Rao R, Saint-Cyr M, Ma AM, et al. Prediction of postoperative necrosis after mastectomy: a pilot study utilizing optical diffusion imaging spectroscopy. World J Surg Oncol 2009;7:91.

52. Saint-Cyr M, Wong C, Schaverien M, et al. The perforasome theory: vascular anatomy and clinical implications. Plast Reconstr Surg 2009;124:1529.

Assessing Perforator Architecture

Michel Saint-Cyr, MD, FRCS(C)

KEYWORDS

- Flap design • Perforator flaps • Perforasome • TRAM flap
- DIEP flap

Increased knowledge of vascular anatomy has inevitably led to innovations in flap design and use in the clinical arena. The evolution of random-pattern flaps to fasciocutaneous flaps to myocutaneous flaps and finally to perforator flaps has followed a linear progression largely because of the pioneering vascular anatomy work produced by Manchot, Salmon, Cormack, Lamberty, Taylor, Palmer, Morris, and others.[1–6] The information derived from such work has fueled the evolution of flap design and applications clinically. The ultimate goal of reconstruction is to match optimal tissue replacement with minimal donor-site expenditure and maintain function. The evolution of refinements over the last 30 years has allowed flaps to be based on specific perforators.

The perforator flap concept was introduced by Kroll and Rosenfield in 1988[7] in their description of a new type of flap based on unnamed perforators located near the midline of the lower back region for low posterior midline defects. These investigators noted that such flaps combined the superior blood supply of the myocutaneous flap with the lack of donor-site morbidity of a skin flap. The beginning of the perforator flap area was crystallized in 1989 when Koshima and Soeda[8] described an inferior epigastric artery skin flap without rectus abdominis muscle pedicled on the muscle perforators and the proximal inferior deep epigastric artery for the reconstruction of floor of the mouth and groin defects. These investigators noted that a large flap without muscle could survive on a single muscle perforator, and the perforator flap era had begun.

The benefits of perforator flaps have been widely published in the literature, and these include decreased donor-site morbidity with decreased postoperative pain and narcotic use.[9–13] The underlying muscle is preserved, often leading to faster recovery and the ability to tailor the flap to reconstruct exactly the tissues that are missing at the recipient site. Musculocutaneous flaps tend to cause bulkiness at the recipient site and when denervated may atrophy at an unpredictable rate, leading to poor aesthetic results. A perforator flap may also be thinned either as a 1-stage or as a 2-stage procedure, allowing contouring of shallow defects that is not possible with a musculocutaneous flap. There is also freedom of orientation of the pedicle, and a longer pedicle than can be achieved with the parent musculocutaneous flap. Although the learning curve may be steeper and dissection more delicate, many agree that perforator flaps have benefits that outweigh the risks.

METHODS OF STUDYING VASCULAR ANATOMY

Flaps were harvested from fresh cadavers from the University of Texas Willed Body Program. Types of flaps included deep inferior epigastric artery perforator (DIEP), superior gluteal artery perforator flap (SGAP), and thoracodorsal artery perforator (TDAP) flaps.[14–17] These were injected with contrast to determine the vascular territory in the zones of perfusion. All flaps were then submitted to static and dynamic computed tomography (CT) scan imaging.

Dynamic (Four-dimensional) CT Scanning

Dynamic or four-dimensional (4D) CT scanning refers to sequential images produced by repeated

Department of Plastic Surgery, University of Texas Southwestern Medical Center at Dallas, 1801 Inwood Road, Dallas, TX 75390-9132, USA
E-mail address: michel.saint-cyr@utsouthwestern.edu

Clin Plastic Surg 38 (2011) 175–202
doi:10.1016/j.cps.2011.03.015
0094-1298/11/$ – see front matter. Published by Elsevier Inc.

scanning as contrast flows through the flap. This technique results in a video of simulated flap perfusion. Single perforator injections were performed with iodinated contrast medium and the flap subjected to dynamic CT scanning using a GE Lightspeed 16-slice scanner (General Electric, Milwaukee, WI, USA). Scans were repeated at timed intervals, thus giving us progressive CT images over time. We found a total volume of 3 to 4 mL of contrast was sufficient for each flap injection.

Static (Three-dimensional) CT Scanning

A barium-gelatin mixture was injected into the investigated perforator to fill the vascular territory. Flaps were then frozen for at least 24 hours before CT scanning.

Three-dimensional (3D) and 4D images were viewed using the TeraRecon Aquarius workstation (version 3.2.2.21; TeraRecon, Inc, San Mateo, CA, USA). The volume-rendering function allowed us to produce clear and accurate images of the simulated flaps.

THE PERFORASOME, DIRECT, AND INDIRECT LINKING VESSELS

Each cutaneous perforator has its own unique vascular arterial territory, which we described as being an arterial perforasome.[18] Each perforasome is linked with adjacent perforasomes via 2 main mechanisms. These mechanisms include both direct and indirect linking vessels (**Fig. 1**).

Direct linking vessels are large vessels, which allow flow from 1 perforator to the next and allow the capture of adjacent perforasomes through an interperforator flow mechanism. Large filling pressures or perfusion pressures through a single perforator can allow for large perforator flap harvests such as the extended anterolateral thigh

flap. The linking vessels connect multiple perforasomes to one another (**Fig. 2**).

Perforasomes are also linked to one another by indirect linking vessels or recurrent flow via the subdermal plexus (**Fig. 3**). These vessels are similar to choke vessels described by Taylor.[3] In reality, perforators give off oblique and direct oblique branches to the subdermal plexus, and recurrent flow from the subdermal plexus to an adjacent perforator oblique branch allows capture of an adjacent perforasome via recurrent flow.

These 2 mechanisms of flow are protective mechanisms to ensure vascular connection between adjacent perforasomes.

PERFORASOME THEORY
First Principle

Each perforasome is linked with adjacent perforasomes by means of 2 main mechanisms that include both direct and indirect linking vessels.

Second Principle

Flap design and skin paddle orientation should be based on the direction of the linking vessels, which is axial in the extremities and perpendicular to the midline in the trunk. Orientation of the linking vessels corresponds to the orientation of maximal blood flow, and flap axis should ideally be designed to respect this.

Third Principle

Preferential filling of perforasomes occurs within perforators of the same source artery first, followed by perforators of other adjacent source arteries. Vascular filling and density are maximized in the periphery of the perforasome within the same source artery. The linking vessels then emanate from this main perforasome to perforasomes

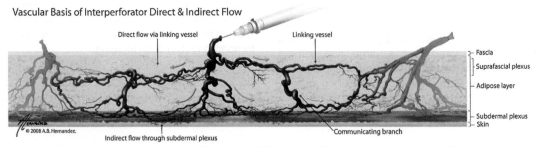

Vascular Basis of Interperforator Direct & Indirect Flow

Direct flow via linking vessel   Linking vessel

Fascia
Suprafascial plexus
Adipose layer
Subdermal plexus
Skin

© 2008 A.B. Hernandez.   Indirect flow through subdermal plexus   Communicating branch

Fig. 1. Interperforator flow occurs by means of direct and indirect linking vessels. Direct linking vessels communicate directly with an adjacent perforator to maintain perfusion, and travel within the suprafascial and adipose tissue layers. Indirect linking vessels communicate with adjacent perforators by means of recurrent flow through the subdermal plexus. Communicating branches between direct and indirect linking vessels are also seen and help maintain vascular perfusion in case of injury. (Printed with permission from A.B. Hernandez of Gory Details Illustration, Grapevine, TX.)

PERFUSION IN MULTIPLE PERFORASOMES VIA LINKING VESSELS

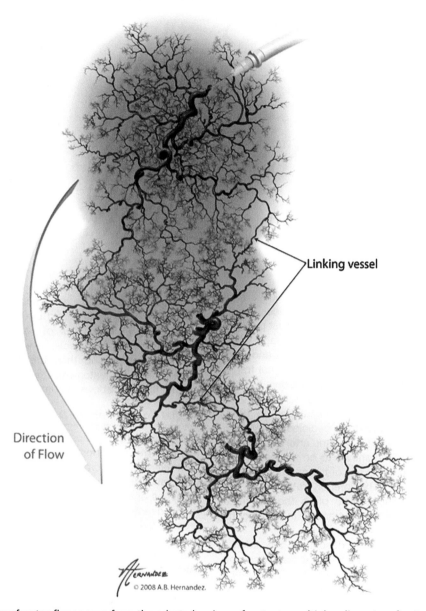

Linking vessel

Direction of Flow

© 2008 A.B. Hernandez.

Fig. 2. Interperforator flow occurs from the selected main perforator to multiple adjacent perforators by means of direct linking vessels and indirect linking vessels (recurrent flow from subdermal plexus). High perfusion pressures through the main perforator open multiple direct and indirect linking vessels and allow perfusion of multiple other perforasomes. In this way, large flaps such as the anterolateral thigh flap can be harvested based on a single perforator. (Printed with permission from A.B. Hernandez of Gory Details Illustration, Grapevine, TX.)

of adjacent vascular territories from other source arteries.

Fourth Principle

Mass vascularity of a perforator found adjacent to an articulation is directed away from that same articulation (eg, distally and proximally based radial artery perforator flaps), whereas perforators found at a midpoint between 2 articulations (eg, upper extremity) or at the midpoint in the trunk have a multidirectional flow distribution. Therefore, flap design should take into consideration perforator location.[18]

INDIRECT FLOW THROUGH THE SUBDERMAL PLEXUS

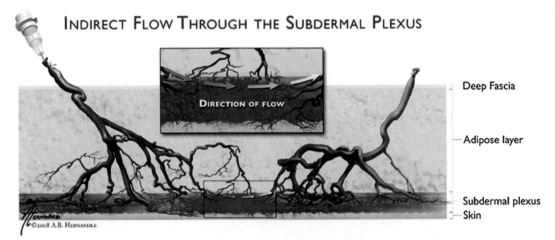

DIRECTION OF FLOW

Deep Fascia

Adipose layer

Subdermal plexus
Skin

©2008 A.B. HERNANDEZ

Fig. 3. Lateral view of an indirect linking vessel that maintains perfusion from 1 perforator to the next by means of recurrent flow from the subdermal plexus. (Printed with permission from A.B. Hernandez of Gory Details Illustration, Grapevine, TX.)

DIEP FLAP

Use of abdominal tissue for autologous breast reconstruction has been long and widely practiced. It is an ideal source, because most patients who develop breast cancer are at an age when they also have excessive abdominal fat and skin. The DIEP flap evolved from the traditional transverse rectus abdominis myocutaneous (TRAM) flap. Holstrom first described the free (TRAM) flap in 1979[19] for breast reconstruction. In 1982, Hartrampf[20] popularized the pedicled TRAM flap, based on the superior epigastric artery. However, this artery has been shown to be the secondary blood supply to the tissue of the anterior abdominal wall.[17–19,21,22] The inferior, rather than the superior, epigastric pedicle plays the dominant role in abdominal tissue transfer in autologous breast reconstruction.

Koshima and Soeda described the inferior epigastric artery skin flap,[23] but it was Allen and Treece[24] who first used the DIEP flap for breast reconstruction, which has now become common practice in many plastic surgical units.

Anatomy

Like a free TRAM flap, the pedicle of the DIEP flap is the deep inferior epigastric artery (DIEA), which originates from the medial aspect of the external iliac artery just above the inguinal ligament. The DIEA is the most significant artery supplying the skin of the anterior abdominal wall, with a pedicle 7.5 to 20.5 cm long and 3.3 0.4 mm in diameter with 2 accompanying venae commitantes in most cases.[25] There are 52 perforators from the DIEA concentrated in the periumbilical region. It forms 2 main intramuscular branches in most

cases: the lateral branch, which gives a lateral row of perforators in the lateral third of the muscle, communicating through deep anastomoses with the lower 4 intercostals; and the medial branch, which gives a medial row of perforators in the medial third of the muscle, which gives off an umbilical branch and then terminates in deep choke vessel anastomoses with the superior epigastric artery above the umbilicus.

Medial Row Perforator DIEP Flap

In our study of DIEP flaps, the mean vascular territory for a medial perforator DIEP flap injected with contrast was 296 cm^2 ($P<.008$ when compared with vascular territory of lateral perforator). The branches of the medial row perforator were seen to be directed both laterally and medially, and crossed the midline in all cases. The vascular territories of these flaps were more centralized compared with those perfused by a lateral perforator (**Fig. 4**). Large-diameter linking vessels were found to connect perforators within the same medial row (**Fig. 5**). The injected medial perforators connected with contralateral medial row perforators (across the midline) through the indirect linking vessels via the subdermal plexus (**Figs. 6** and **7**). Moon and Taylor[26] also noted that crossover of the midline is predominantly in the subdermal plexus. Medial row and lateral row perforators within the same hemiabdomen were connected via both direct and indirect linking vessels (see **Fig. 7**).

When planning a large breast reconstruction, a medial row perforator or a combination of medial and lateral perforators (muscle-sparing TRAM or TRAM flap) should be considered. If a single medial row perforator is selected, the vascular

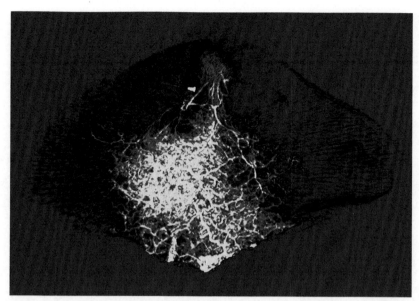

Fig. 4. Anteroposterior view of an abdominal adipocutaneous flap where the whole abdominal skin was harvested, bordered by the costal margins, midaxillary lines (*MAL*), and pubis. A single dominant medial perforator was injected with contrast. Perfusion extends to zones I, II, and III, the level of the pubis, and almost to the left costal margin.

territory is larger, and more centralized, compared with a lateral row perforator-based flap. Therefore, both tips of the flap are the furthest away from the medial perforator and are subjected to a higher risk of ischemia (**Fig. 8**). When selecting a perforator for DIEP flap surgery, the largest perforator should be selected. We found in both clinical and cadaver dissections that periumbilical perforators were the most dominant/largest perforators in most cases (**Fig. 9**).

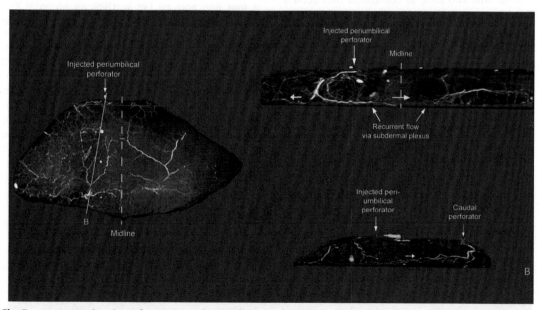

Fig. 5. nteroposterior view of a transverse lower abdominal adipocutaneous flap where a single dominant medial perforator was injected with contrast. (*Above, right*) Transverse view of flap, corresponding to line A. Perfusion crosses the midline by means of the subdermal plexus. (*Below, right*) Sagittal view of flap, corresponding to line B. X marks a perforator caudal to the injected periumbilical one. Yellow arrows show direction of flow.

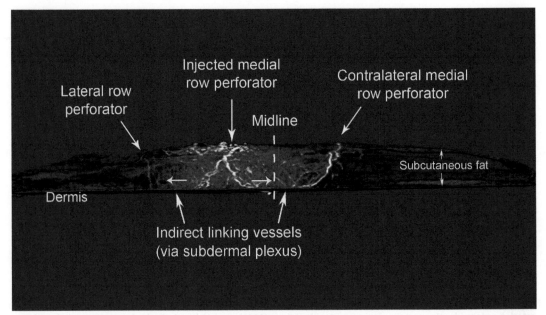

Fig. 6. 3D CT angiogram of a medial perforator DIEP flap, transverse view. The injected medial perforator was connected to the contralateral medial row perforator through indirect linking vessels via the subdermal plexus. The yellow arrows show the direction of flow.

In our 4D CT investigations, we found that flow of contrast for a medial perforator DIEP traveled earlier to zone II and had a greater area of vascularity compared with zone III (**Fig. 10**). The lateral perforator DIEP flaps had earlier and greater contrast flow into zone III compared with zone II (**Fig. 11**).

SINGLE DOMINANT MEDIAL ROW PERFORATOR DIEP FLAP

The single dominant perforator DIEP flap is based on a single medial row perforator, which was first described by Koshima and colleagues as a free flap and by Lin in 1989 as an axial flap (**Figs. 12–24**).[23,27] Recent studies discussing the

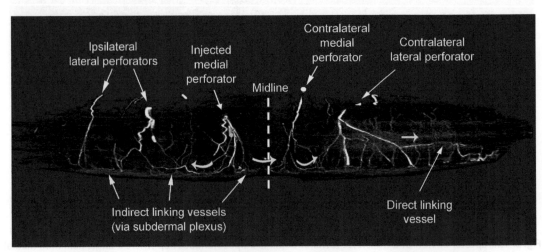

Fig. 7. 3D CT scan of a lower abdominal adipocutaneous flap where a single dominant medial perforator was injected with contrast (transverse view). Flow between adjacent perforators is through indirect linking vessels (by means of the subdermal plexus) or direct linking vessels. Yellow arrows show direction of flow.

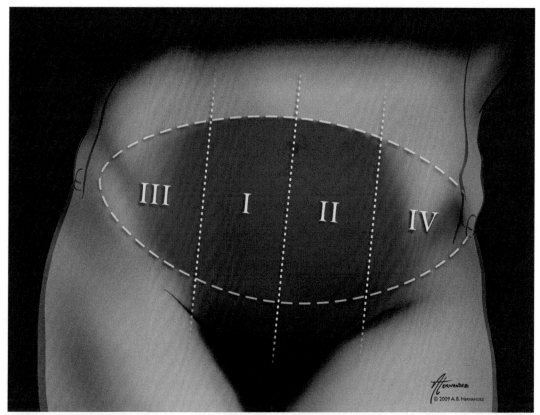

Fig. 8. A medial perforator DIEP flap, in which perfusion is more centralized and has a bigger vascular territory. These flaps are useful for large breast reconstructions. (Printed with permission from A.B. Hernandez of Gory Details Illustration, Grapevine, TX.)

dominance of the lateral versus the medial row perforators have shown dominance of the medial row perforators over the lateral row perforators. To determine the location and vascularity of the most dominant medial row perforator in the lower abdomen we recently conducted a clinical and anatomic study looking at outcomes such as perforator size, location, and type; zones of

Fig. 9. Single dominant medial perforator location. The red dots indicate the individual perforator locations and the black dots represent the average perforator locations.

perfusion were documented for all flaps and clinical outcomes for all patients.

In a recent study at our institution, 11 abdominal flaps were harvested from fresh adult cadavers, and measurements were combined with clinical measurements from 16 patients. A total of 36 flaps were dissected, with an average perforator location within a 3-cm radius of the umbilicus and an average perforator size greater than 1.8 mm. CT scans of the cadaver abdominal flaps showed consistent perfusion in zones I and II and half of zones III and IV.

Clinical results showed partial flap necrosis in 1 patient and fat necrosis of less than 5% in 3 patients, all of which occurred in the distal portion of zone III. The DIEA medial row perforators near the umbilicus were found to be the largest perforators in the entire DIEA system and abdomen (see **Fig. 9**).

The single dominant medial row perforator has a maximal vascularity in zones I and II, and less in zones III and IV. Based on this study we recommend that half of zone III and all of zone IV be discarded to avoid the risks of partial flap loss and fat

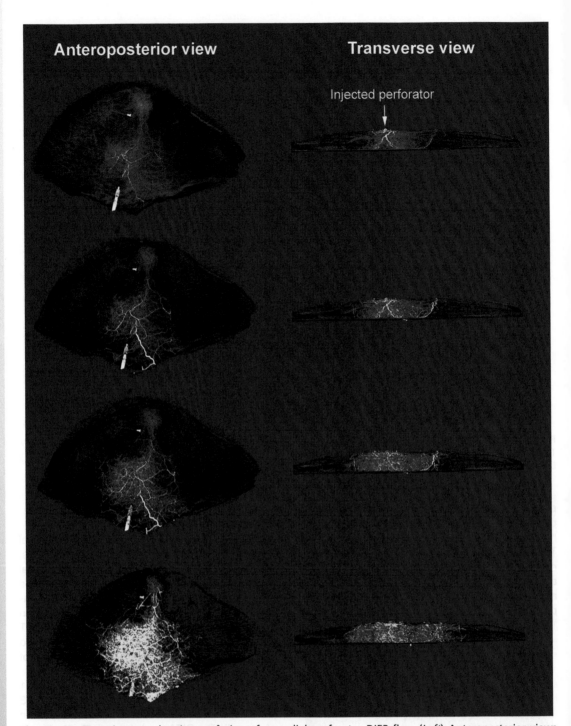

Anteroposterior view

Transverse view

Injected perforator

Fig. 10. 4D CT angiograms showing perfusion of a medial perforator DIEP flap. (*Left*) Anteroposterior views. (*Right*) Transverse views. Flow of contrast traveled earlier to zone II and had a greater area of vascularity compared with zone III.

necrosis. Flap vascularity should also be evaluated intraoperatively and all zones that show signs of venous congestion or marginal arterial perfusion need to be discarded.

LATERAL ROW PERFORATOR DIEP FLAP

Lateral row perforators are simple to harvest and when found close to the lateral edge of the rectus muscle, they follow a more direct vertical

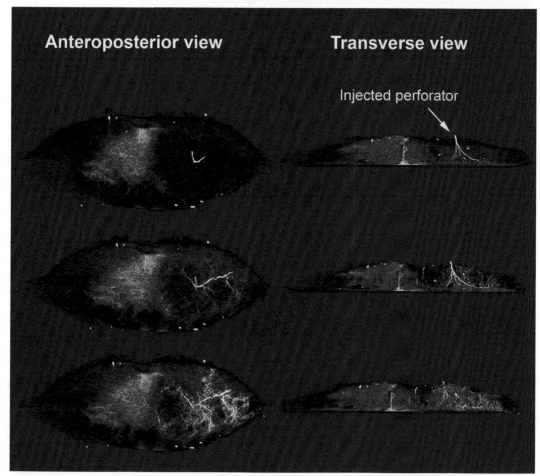

Fig. 11. 4D CT angiograms showing perfusion of a lateral perforator DIEP flap. (*Left*) Anteroposterior views. (*Right*) Transverse views. There was earlier and greater contrast flow into zone III compared with zone II.

orientation when passing through the muscle to the lateral division of the DIEA and vein. Studies have been performed that advocate the use of the lateral row perforators in DIEP flap harvesting. The lateral branch is frequently wider, and tends to run a more rectilinear course, allowing for easier and speedier dissection.[28,29]

In our study, the mean vascular territory of a DIEP flap when a lateral row perforator was injected was 196 cm^2, which is smaller than a medial perforator DIEP. Perfusion was found to be more lateralized, and few of these flaps crossed the midline. Contrast injected into a lateral perforator tended to stay in 1 hemiabdomen. This result was likely to be because of a higher number of communicating vessels needed to cross the midline, compared with a flap based on a medial perforator (**Fig. 25**).

Large-diameter linking vessels were found to connect perforators within the same lateral row

perforators, and both direct and indirect linking vessels were found to communicate between perforators of the same hemiabdomen (**Fig. 26**).

Lateral row perforators used in a hemiabdominal flap have more of a central position, and have less risk of partial flap necrosis of the most distal ipsilateral tip of the flap. Therefore, hemiabdominal flaps tend to be safely harvested based off a single lateral row perforator (**Fig. 27**), and this can be used in small to medium breast reconstructions. It is also useful for bilateral breast reconstruction.

DIEP FLAP AND REAPPRAISAL OF THE ZONES OF PERFUSION

Holm and colleagues performed vascular perfusion studies, which demonstrated that Hartrampf zones II and III should be reversed.[30] These investigators noted that perfusion of the vascular territories across the midline was always delayed and

Single Dominant Medial Perforator DIEP Flap
Type I (Intramuscular)

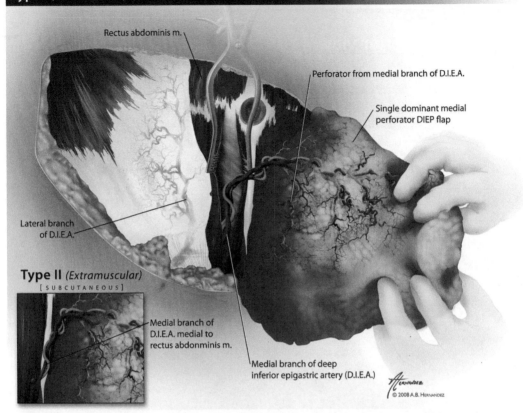

Rectus abdominis m.

Perforator from medial branch of D.I.E.A.

Single dominant medial perforator DIEP flap

Lateral branch of D.I.E.A.

Type II (Extramuscular)
[S U B C U T A N E O U S]

Medial branch of D.I.E.A. medial to rectus abdonminis m.

Medial branch of deep inferior epigastric artery (D.I.E.A.)

© 2008 A.B. Hernandez

Fig. 12. The underside of a harvested single dominant medial perforator DIEP flap. Inset shows alternate path of medial branch of the deep inferior epigastric artery (type II or extramuscular single dominant medial perforator). (Printed with permission from A.B. Hernandez of Gory Details Illustration, Grapevine, TX.)

Single Dominant Medial Perforator DIEP Flap Anatomy
Type I (Intramuscular)

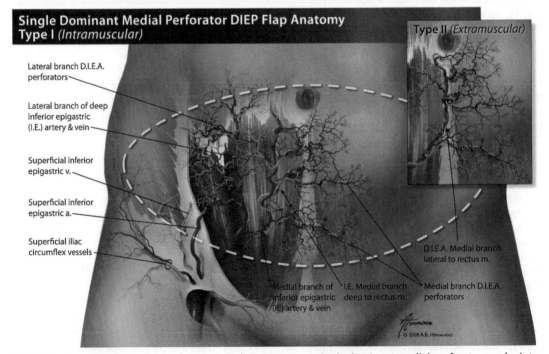

Type II (Extramuscular)

Lateral branch D.I.E.A. perforators

Lateral branch of deep inferior epigastric (I.E.) artery & vein

Superficial inferior epigastric v.

Superficial inferior epigastric a.

Superficial iliac circumflex vessels

D.I.E.A. Medial branch lateral to rectus m.

Medial branch of inferior epigastric (IE) artery & vein

I.E. Medial branch deep to rectus m.

Medial branch D.I.E.A. perforators

© 2008 A.B. Hernandez

Fig. 13. Single dominant medial perforator DIEP flap anatomy. A single dominant medial perforator can be intramuscular (type I) or extramuscular (type II), as shown in the inset. (Printed with permission from A.B. Hernandez of Gory Details Illustration, Grapevine, TX.)

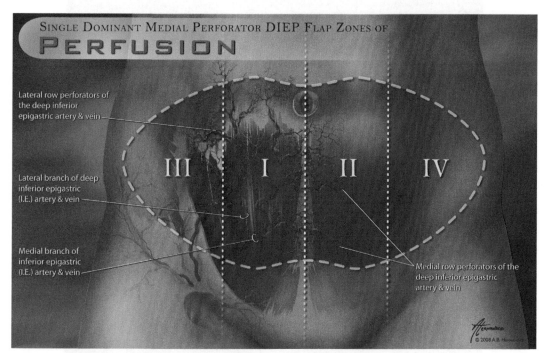

Fig. 14. Single dominant medial perforator DIEP flap zones of perfusion. (Printed with permission from A.B. Hernandez of Gory Details Illustration, Grapevine, TX.)

less intensive than in the territories on the ipsilateral side. In Holm and colleagues' study, only 2 of 15 flaps used only the medial row perforators, and 8 used only lateral row perforators (the rest had both medial and lateral row perforators).

Based on our previous 3D and 4D CT angiographic studies, contrast flow from a medial perforator perfused Hartrampf zone II earlier and more so than Hartrampf zone III. The resultant area of vascularity of Hartrampf zone II is greater than in Hartrampf zone III. Therefore, flaps based on a single medial row perforator are shown to be more centralized, and follow Hartrampf's classification of perfusion zones, with zone II being the

contralateral medial region of a transverse abdominal flap. Zone III is ipsilateral to zone I and zone IV is ipsilateral to zone II (**Fig. 28**).

In contrast, perfusion for a lateral perforator DIEP is more lateralized. Contrast traveled to Hartrampf zone III earlier and had a greater area of vascularity compared with Hartrampf zone II. Therefore, this perfusion pattern follows Holm's classification, and zones II and III should be in reverse order (**Fig. 29**). Holm zone II corresponds to the area ipsilateral to zone I, and Holm zone III should now be the contralateral medial region, in the same hemiabdomen as zone IV (**Fig. 30**).

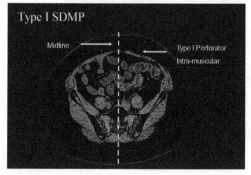

Fig. 15. Type I (intramuscular) single dominant medial perforator shown on a patient's CT angiogram.

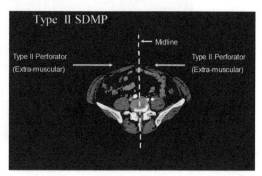

Fig. 16. Type II (extramuscular) single dominant medial perforator shown on a patient's CT angiogram.

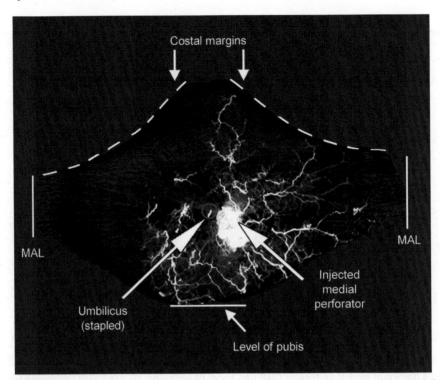

Fig. 17. Anteroposterior view of an abdominal adipocutaneous flap where the whole abdominal skin was harvested, bordered by the costal margins, midaxillary lines (*MAL*), and pubis. A single dominant medial perforator was injected with contrast. Perfusion extends to zones I, II, and III, the level of the pubis, and almost to the left costal margin.

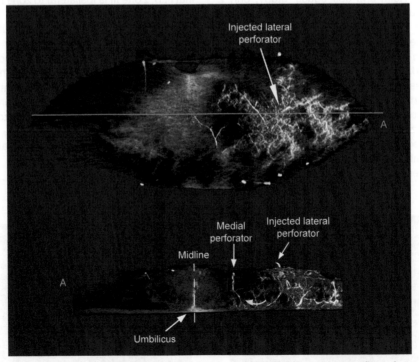

Fig. 18. (*Above*) Anteroposterior view of a transverse lower abdominal adipocutaneous flap where a lateral row perforator was injected with contrast. Note that only the hemiabdomen (zones I and III) is perfused. (*Below*) Transverse view of the flap, corresponding to line A. Perfusion extends to an adjacent medial perforator but not across the midline. Yellow arrow shows direction of flow.

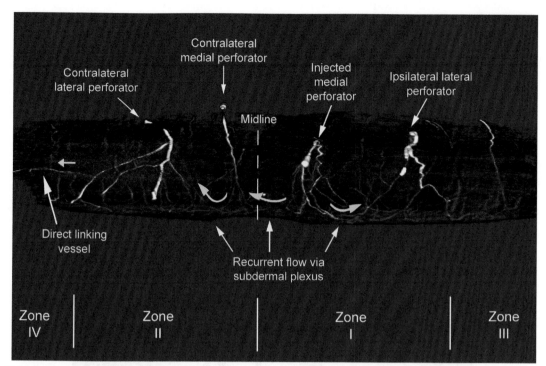

Fig. 19. 3D CT scan of a lower abdominal adipocutaneous flap where a single dominant medial perforator was injected with contrast (transverse view). Flow between adjacent perforators is through indirect linking vessels (by means of the subdermal plexus) or direct linking vessels. Yellow arrows show direction of flow.

APPLYING THE PERFORASOME CONCEPT TO DIEP ZONES OF PERFUSION

Perforators each have their own vascular territory (perforasome) and capture adjacent perforasomes via direct and indirect linking vessels. With respect to the DIEP flap, the focus has now shifted from the vascular supply and anatomy of the source artery (DIEA) to the individual perforators themselves. The number of adjacent perforasomes that are perfused via the selected main perforator(s) of a DIEP flap dictates the overall vascular territory and survival of the flaps. All previous classification schemes for the lower abdomen

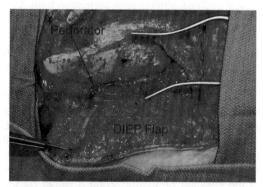

Fig. 20. Type I single dominant medial perforator flap. The intramuscular course of the perforator necessitates splitting of the rectus muscle. Note the long pedicle that can be achieved when a periumbilical perforator is selected. Dissection is stopped at the lateral edge of the rectus muscle or until a sufficient pedicle external diameter is obtained.

Fig. 21. Type II single dominant medial perforator flap. Note the extramuscular course of the perforator medial to the medial border of the rectus muscle. This perforator is found between the linea alba and the medial border of the rectus muscle and therefore can be considered subcutaneous. In all cases, type II perforators represented the terminal branch of the medial division of the deep inferior epigastric artery and vein to the umbilicus.

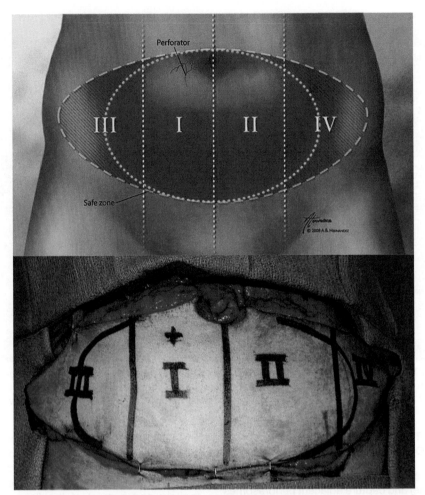

Fig. 22. (*Above*) Safe zones of the single dominant medial perforator DIEP flap are illustrated by the blue dotted line. The lateral portion of zone III and all of zone IV are routinely discarded. (*Below*) Single dominant medial perforator DIEP flap harvested on a single perforator (*X* in zone I), with zones of perfusion and safe zones of harvest outlined. (Printed with permission from A.B. Hernandez of Gory Details Illustration, Grapevine, TX.)

and DIEP flap have been based on the DIEA source vessel vascular territory (angiosome of the DIEA).

Classifying the perfusion of the DIEP flap based on the perforasome of either the medial or lateral row perforator can be described as follows: zone 1 corresponds to the selected perforator itself (medial or lateral row perforator) and zone 2 corresponds to the adjacent perforasome on either side of the selected perforator. Zone 3 would be the second perforasome distal to the selected zone 1 perforator, and so forth.

MEDIAL ROW DIEP PERFORASOME CLASSIFICATION

- Zone 1: perforasome of the medial row perforator (**Fig. 31**)

- Zone 2: first perforasome distal to zone 1: perforasome of ipsilateral lateral row and contralateral medial row
- Zone 3: second perforasome distal to zone 1: perforasome of contralateral lateral row and vascular territory of the ipsilateral superficial inferior epigastric artery (SIEA)
- Zone 4: vascular territory of contralateral SIEA.

LATERAL ROW DIEP PERFORASOME CLASSIFICATION

- Zone 1: perforasome of the lateral row perforator (**Fig. 32**)
- Zone 2: first perforasome distal to zone 1: perforasome of ipsilateral medial row and vascular territory of the ipsilateral SIEA

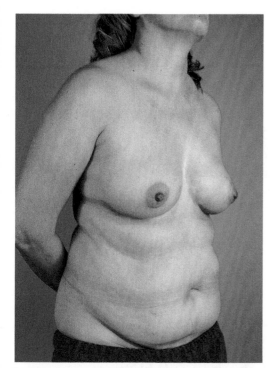

Fig. 23. Preoperative image of a 38-year-old woman with ductal carcinoma of the right breast.

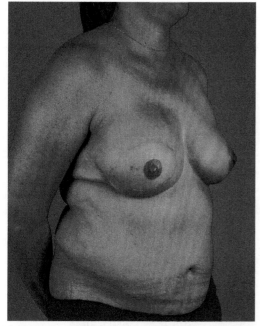

Fig. 24. Postoperative view at 6 months after right breast skin-sparing mastectomy and immediate reconstruction with a single dominant medial perforator DIEP flap, and 4 months after nipple reconstruction using a C-V flap.

- Zone 3: second perforasome distal to zone 1: perforasome of contralateral medial row
- Zone 4: third perforasome distal to zone 1: perforasome of contralateral lateral row
- Zone 5: vascular territory of contralateral SIEA.

SAFE AND UNSAFE ZONES OF DIEP FLAP HARVEST
Medial Row DIEP

- 2,1,2: very reliable
- 3*,2,1: very reliable (* one-third or half of zone 3 discarded)
- 3*,2,1,2: reliable
- 3*,2,1,2,3: variable
- 3*,2,1,2,3,4: variable.

Lateral Row DIEP

- 2,1,2: very reliable
- 2,1,2,3: variable
- 2,1,2,3,4: less reliable
- 2,1,2,3,4,5: much less reliable.

TDAP FLAP

The TDAP flap (**Fig. 33**) was first described by Angrigiani and colleagues[31] in 1995, when they reported raising the cutaneous island of the latissimus dorsi musculocutaneous flap without muscle based on only 1 cutaneous perforator. The TDAP flap has a few known disadvantages. It has been accused of having anatomic inconsistency of the perforators, as well as the difficulty of having a 2-team approach. However, the TDAP flap is a safe and versatile flap with a long pedicle and a large flap dimension of up to 25 × 15 cm as reported by Angrigiani and colleagues, which was closed primarily. The donor site is aesthetically acceptable and preserves the function of the underlying latissimus dorsi muscle without producing a seroma. For a sensate flap a lateral branch of the intercostal nerve can be included in the flap. Besides being used as a pedicled flap in breast reconstruction, it is also indicated in head and neck reconstruction and trunk reconstruction. As a free flap, it can be used for reconstruction of traumatic upper and lower extremity defects, including the possibility of use as a flow-through flap. Donor sites up to 10 cm wide can be closed primarily.

Anatomy

The flap derives its blood supply from the perforating vessels that originate from the descending and transverse branch of the thoracodorsal artery. The descending branch is known to have the

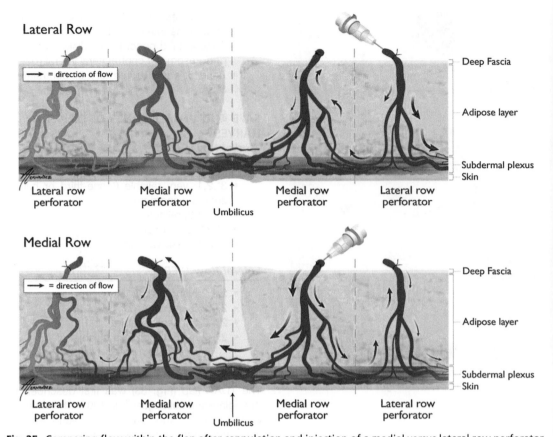

Fig. 25. Comparing flow within the flap after cannulation and injection of a medial versus lateral row perforator (lateral view). Note that in the lateral row perforator, flow predominantly occurs laterally, with perfusion not seen to extend beyond the contralateral medial row perforator after passing through the subdermal plexus twice. The medial row perforators are connected across the midline by large-diameter linking vessels, with flap perfusion up to the contralateral lateral row perforators. (Printed with permission from A.B. Hernandez of Gory Details Illustration, Grapevine, TX.)

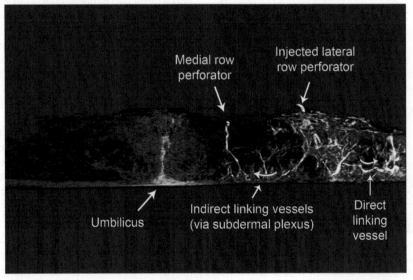

Fig. 26. Transverse view of the flap. Perfusion extends to an adjacent medial perforator but not across the midline. Yellow arrow shows direction of flow.

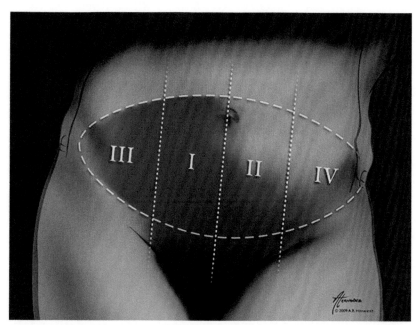

Fig. 27. Vascularity of predominantly the lateral row perforators showing good vascularity of the ipsilateral hemiabdomen. (Printed with permission from A.B. Hernandez of Gory Details Illustration, Grapevine, TX.)

largest and most reliable perforating vessels, and is found descending along a line at approximately 2 cm behind the anterior border of the latissimus dorsi muscle edge.[32] In the original flap description Angrigiani and colleagues[31] found that the descending branch provided 2 to 3 perforators, with the proximal perforator found approximately 8 cm below the posterior axillary fold and 2 to 3 cm from the lateral border of the muscle, with distal perforators spaced 2 to 4 cm apart.

Perforators located close to the hilus of the thoracodorsal artery are reliable in presence and size.

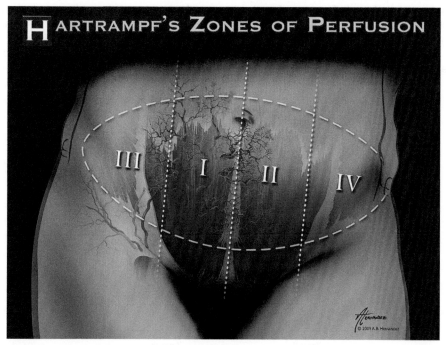

Fig. 28. Hartrampf zones of perfusion. (Printed with permission from A.B. Hernandez of Gory Details Illustration, Grapevine, TX.)

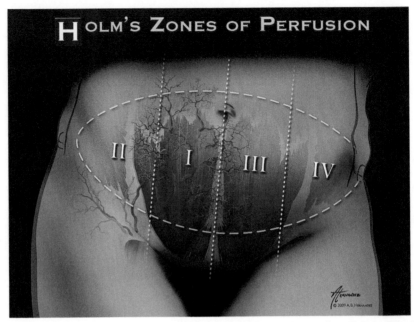

Fig. 29. Holm zones of perfusion. (Printed with permission from A.B. Hernandez of Gory Details Illustration, Grapevine, TX.)

The first perforator is usually the largest and most consistent. Thomas and colleagues[32] in a study of 15 fresh cadavers noted that there were a mean of 5.5 perforators for each specimen, with musculocutaneous perforators predominating, which were seen to penetrate the latissimus dorsi muscle in its cephalad third. The mean length of the pedicle was 14 cm, with a 2.8 mm diameter at the origin. At least 2 musculocutaneous perforators were noted approximately 3 cm from the anterior border of the muscle, the most proximal being at the level of the inferior angle of the scapula. Septocutaneous perforators from the thoracodorsal artery supplying the skin in addition to the musculocutaneous perforators were seen in 60% of specimens.

In our study of the TDAP flap,[16] in all specimens, the thoracodorsal artery bifurcated into transverse and descending branches at the neurovascular hilus at a mean distance of 5.1 cm (range 2.1–7.5 cm) from the posterior axillary fold, 2.2 cm (range 1.3–3.1) from the lateral edge of the latissimus

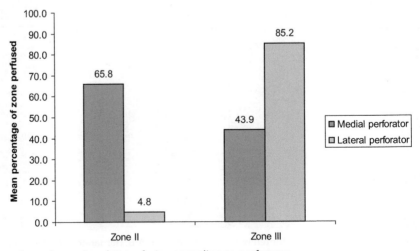

Fig. 30. Comparison of zone II and III perfusion according to perforator.

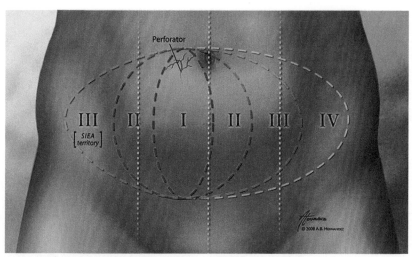

Fig. 31. Perforasome of a single medial DIEA perforator. The perforasome of the medial perforator corresponds to zone I and every adjacent perforasome is equivalent to zone II, zone III, and so forth (Zone II: ipsilateral lateral row perforator, and contralateral medial row perforator. Every adjacent perforasome to the second perforator is zone III and so forth.). (Printed with permission from A.B. Hernandez of Gory Details Illustration, Grapevine, TX.)

dorsi muscle. A mean of 3.6 musculocutaneous perforators (range 1 to 8) of 0.5 mm were found per flap, with 70% originating from the descending branch, and perforators from the transverse branch found in 66% of flaps. At least 1 perforator originated from the descending branch in all dissections. A second perforator was observed in 12 (80%) dissections, a third in 5 (33%), and a fourth in 3 (20%) specimens (**Fig. 34**). The most proximal perforator from the descending branch was noted to have the largest diameter in all specimens, except one, where the second perforator was noted to have the largest diameter. In addition, a direct extramuscular branch from the thoracodorsal artery was observed coursing over the lateral edge of the muscle giving rise to a septocutaneous perforator. This was noted in 8 of 15 dissections (53%).

In 3D and 4D CT scanning cadaver TDAP flaps, we found that perfusion occurred through direct and indirect linking vessels, similar to the DIEP flap (**Figs. 35–37**).

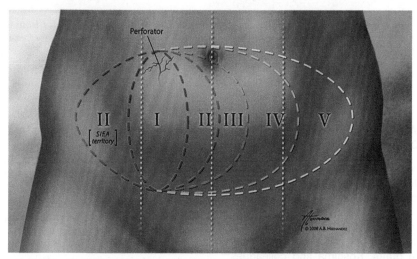

Fig. 32. Same perfusion principle as in **Fig. 31**. The lateral row perforator vascularizes the hemiabdomen by capturing additional adjacent perforators (perforasomes). (Printed with permission from A.B. Hernandez of Gory Details Illustration, Grapevine, TX.)

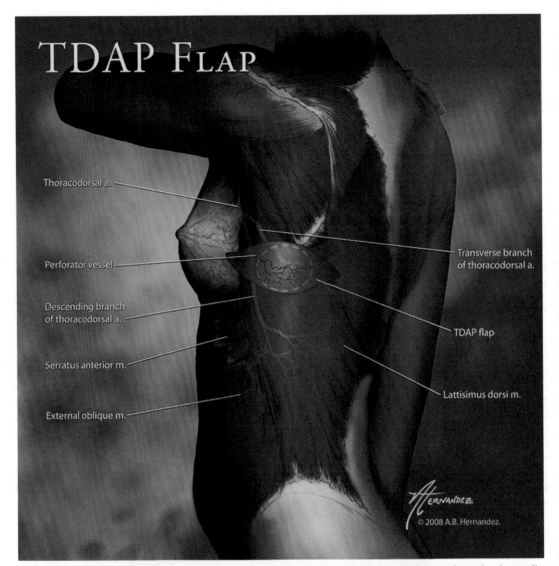

TDAP FLAP

Thoracodorsal a.

Perforator vessel

Descending branch
of thoracodorsal a.

Serratus anterior m.

External oblique m.

Transverse branch
of thoracodorsal a.

TDAP flap

Lattisimus dorsi m.

ERNANDEZ
© 2008 A.B. Hernandez.

Fig. 33. Vascular anatomy of the thoracodorsal artery perforator flap based on a perforator from the descending branch of the thoracodorsal artery (Printed with permission from A.B. Hernandez of Gory Details Illustration, Grapevine, TX.).

SUPERIOR AND INFERIOR GLUTEAL ARTERY PERFORATOR FLAPS

Fujino and colleagues[33] described the use of the superior gluteal musculocutaneous flap for breast reconstruction in 1975, and Le-Quang described the inferior gluteal musculocutaneous flap in 1978.[34] The main weaknesses included significant donor-site morbidity, and a short pedicle that often required vein grafts. Koshima and colleagues[35] first described the use of the gluteal artery perforator flap, based on parasacral perforators, for

management of sacral pressure sores. In 1993 Allen and Tucker[36] described the superior gluteal artery perforator (SGAP) flap for breast reconstruction. Since its introduction and that of the inferior gluteal artery perforator (IGAP) flap, many investigators have advocated their use as a first-line alternative for breast reconstruction when the DIEP flap is not available, such as in patients with insufficient abdominal fatty tissue volume, abdominal incisions, or after previous abdominoplasty. Advantages include low donor-site morbidity, a longer vascular pedicle than that of

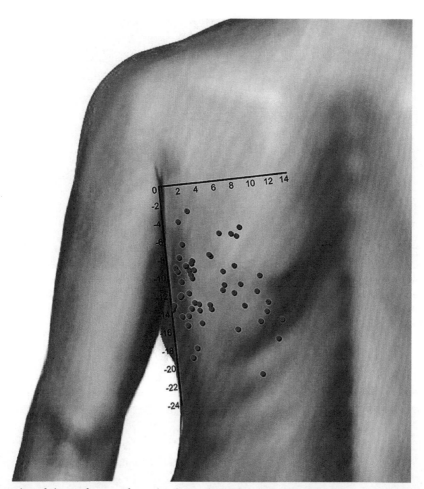

Fig. 34. Scatterplot of the perforators from the descending (*red*) and transverse (*blue*) branches of the thoraco-dorsal artery with respect to the posterior axillary fold. The yellow area represents the region in which the most proximal, and largest, perforator from the descending branch was found in all specimens. This area was found within 3 cm of the lateral edge of the latissimus muscle from 6.6 to 15.4 cm caudal to the posterior axillary fold. A mean of 3.6 musculocutaneous perforators (range 1–8) were found, with a mean of 2.5 (range 1–7) originating from the descending branch and 1.1 (range 0–3) originating from the transverse branch. The mean intramuscular length of perforators was 2.8 cm (range 1.3–4.7 cm) from the descending branch and 3.1 cm (range 1.2–6 cm) for the transverse branch (Printed with permission from A.B. Hernandez of Gory Details Illustration, Grapevine, TX.).

its musculocutaneous predecessor, abundance of adipose tissue even in thin patients, a hidden scar, and good projection of the reconstructed breast.

However, many investigators regard these flaps as the most technically challenging of the options in the armamentarium of the breast reconstructive surgeon. A flap width of up to 13 cm may be closed directly, and the flap length can be up to 30 cm.[37] With the patient placed in the lateral decubitus position 2 teams of surgeons can work simultaneously. There is also potential for sensory reinnervation by anastomosis of the nervi clunium superioris.[38]

Both flaps have their merits and disadvantages. The IGAP flap has the disadvantage of showing a horizontal scar at the level of the gluteal crease, which may not be covered by a bathing suit, as well as the potential risks of injury to the sciatic nerve, and donor-site discomfort when sitting if inadequate fatty protection is left over the bony ischial prominences, especially after bilateral procedures.

However, the SGAP flap can leave unsightly contour abnormalities over the buttock. Guerra and colleagues[39] report that although they initially favored the SGAP because of reduced chances

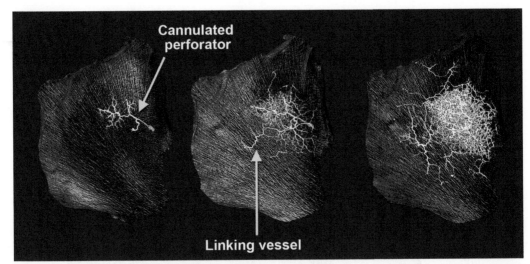

Fig. 35. (*Above*) Anteroposterior dynamic CT angiograms of the most proximal perforator from the descending branch of the thoracodorsal artery at 0.5-mL filling increments. The flap is cut to follow the shape of the latissimus dorsi muscle. Note the large vascular territory and the dense network of linking vessels with the dorsal intercostal artery perforators.

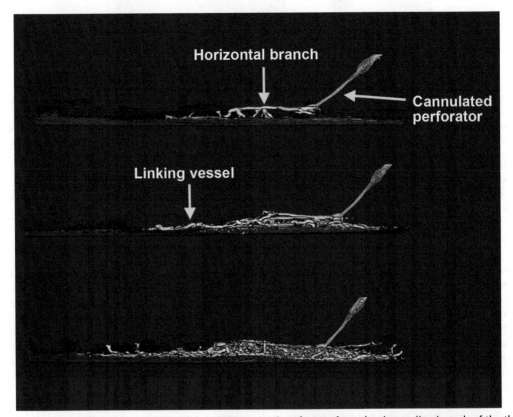

Fig. 36. Lateral dynamic CT angiograms of the most proximal perforator from the descending branch of the thoracodorsal artery at 0.5-mL filling increments. Note that the linking vessels are found deep within the flap at the level of the subdermal plexus, enabling thinning to be performed safely.

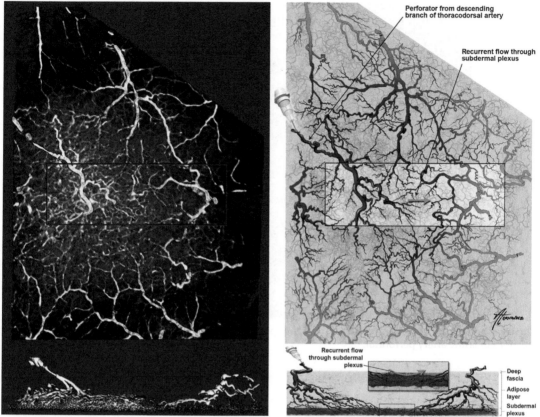

Fig. 37. Static image after cannulation of the most proximal perforator from the descending branch and injection with a barium sulfate/gelatin mixture, with illustration. Note the filling of the adjacent dorsal intercostal artery perforators by means of recurrent flow through the subdermal plexus, with an absence of a suprafascial plexus. This technique enables the flap to be thinned without disrupting its vascular supply (Printed with permission from A.B. Hernandez of Gory Details Illustration, Grapevine, TX.).

of causing paresthesia through injury to the sciatic nerve, they changed their preference to the IGAP when they noted that the flap could be raised without routine exposure of the sciatic nerve and that this flap did not cause some of the contour abnormalities that were seen with the SGAP flaps.[40] For some patients who have excess tissue in the saddlebag area, an IGAP flap may be chosen over an SGAP flap to make use of this extra tissue and provide desirable body contouring.

Anatomy

Both the superior and interior gluteal arteries are terminal branches of the internal iliac artery, leaving the pelvis through the greater sciatic foramen superior and inferior to the piriformis muscle, respectively, with the inferior pedicle accompanied by the greater sciatic nerve and the posterior femoral cutaneous nerve. Koshima

and colleagues[35] noted that 3 perforators usually supply the SGAP cutaneous territory, with a pedicle length of 3 to 8 cm, and 2 to 4 perforators originating from the inferior gluteal artery supply the cutaneous territory of the IGAP flap. The IGAP flap is based on perforators from the inferior gluteal pedicle, and because the course of the inferior gluteal vessels is more oblique through the gluteus maximus muscle than that of the superior gluteal vessels, the length of the IGAP pedicle is longer than that of the SGAP, typically 7 to 10 cm.

In our 3D and 4D CT angiographic investigations, cadaveric SGAP flaps injected with contrast were seen to perfuse almost the whole flap. The midline region received the least amount of contrast (**Fig. 38**). Transverse views showed that like previous flaps, perfusion extended between perforators through recurrent flow via the subdermal plexus of the flap (**Fig. 39**).

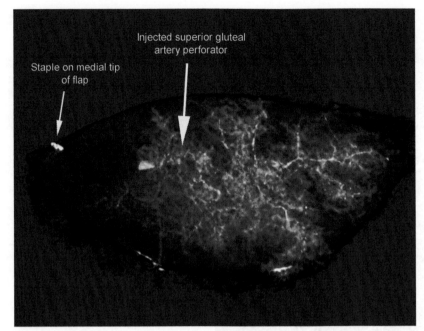

Fig. 38. Anterior view of a superior epigastric artery perforator flap following injection of a single dominant superior epigastric artery perforator.

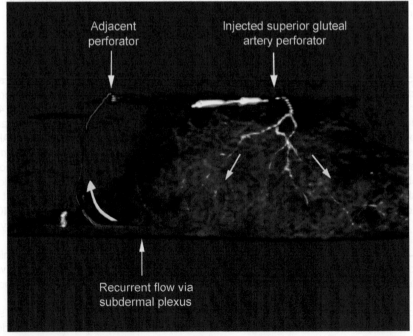

Fig. 39. Lateral view of same SGAP flap as seen in **Fig. 38**. Note interperforator flow via subdermal plexus and also through direct linking vessel, which communicate directly with adjacent perforators.

OTHER PERFORATOR FLAPS
Intercostal Artery Perforator Flaps

The intercostal vessels form an arcade between the aorta and the internal mammary vessels, which gives numerous perforators: dorsal intercostal artery perforator flap, lateral intercostal artery perforator (LICAP) flap, and anterior intercostal artery perforator (AICAP) flap. Every single perforator can be a blood supply to a skin flap. The anatomic studies of Kerrigan and Daniel[41] resulted in a better understanding of the clinical indications and surgical technique of intercostal flaps. Hamdi and colleagues[42] described its use in breast surgery. The intercostal perforators these investigators most commonly used were the ones found anterior to the lateral border of the lastissimus dorsi muscle (LICAP). The pedicle is reported to be merely 4 to 5 cm, but can be increased by dissection within the intercostal muscles. However, this brings with it the risk of creating a pneumothorax.

The LICAP flap is not for whole breast reconstructions. It is indicated for reconstructing breast defects because of its small volume, and only lateral defects at that, because its short pedicle is unable to reach more medial areas (**Figs. 40–43**). For medial defects, the AICAP flap has been reported to be useful.[43]

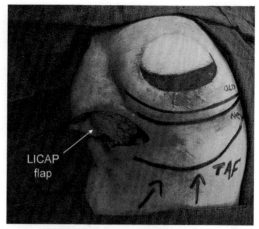

Fig. 41. Intraoperative photograph of LICAP flap being harvested.

Lumbar Artery Perforator Flap

The free lumbar artery perforator flap is a fasciocutaneous flap that was reported to be easy to harvest and leaves an inconspicuous scar (easily hidden by underwear).[44] The axis of the flap passes obliquely from the third lumbar artery to the anterior superior iliac spine. Pedicle length is 4 cm, and the perforators arise between the erector spinae and quadratus lumborum muscles, therefore no intramuscular dissection is necessary. Kato and colleagues[45] performed a fluorescein study showed that the skin territory supplied by the second lumbar artery alone extends from the posterior midline to the lateral border of the

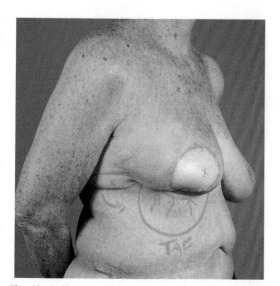

Fig. 40. A 62-year-old patient presented with a defect in the lower outer quadrant of her right breast after free muscle-sparing TRAM reconstruction. Oblique-lateral view of patient, showing markings for LICAP flap (X marks the Dopplered perforator) and thoracoabdominal flap (marked TAF).

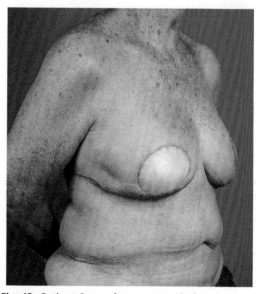

Fig. 42. Patient 6 months postoperatively.

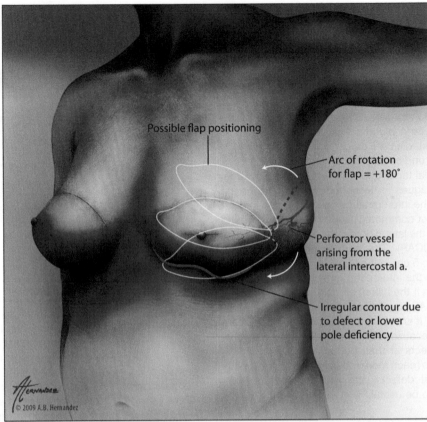

Possible flap positioning

Arc of rotation
for flap = +180°

Perforator vessel
arising from the
lateral intercostal a.

Irregular contour due
to defect or lower
pole deficiency

© 2009 A.B. Hernandez

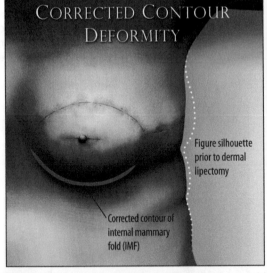

CORRECTED CONTOUR
DEFORMITY

Figure silhouette
prior to dermal
lipectomy

Corrected contour of
internal mammary
fold (IMF)

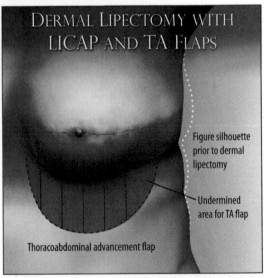

DERMAL LIPECTOMY WITH
LICAP AND TA FLAPS

Figure silhouette
prior to dermal
lipectomy

Undermined
area for TA flap

Thoracoabdominal advancement flap

Fig. 43. *Above:* lower pole breast deformity and possible LICAP flap inset positions. *Bottom left:* corrected lower pole deformity of the breast. Dotted line shows preoperative trunk contour, before dermal lipectomy (LICAP flap harvest). *Bottom right:* correction of lower pole breast deformity with LICAP and thoracoabdominal (TA) flaps (Printed with permission from A.B. Hernandez of Gory Details Illustration, Grapevine, TX.).

rectus sheath and up to 10 cm above the anterior superior iliac spine. Disadvantages of this flap include the need to reposition the patient for breast reconstruction, and patients may notice a slight hypoesthesia in the L1 and L2 dermatomes postoperatively. For cosmetic reasons operative correction of the opposite flank may be necessary at a later date.

SUMMARY

A myriad of options exist for autologous tissue perforator-based breast reconstruction. Each perforator selected has its distinct vascular territory, and proper knowledge of perforator perfusion characteristics helps maximize outcome and limit complications.

REFERENCES

1. Manchot C. The cutaneous arteries of the human body. New York: Springer-Verlag; 1983.
2. Cormack GC, Lamberty BG. Fasciocutaneous vessels. Their distribution on the trunk and limbs, and their clinical application in tissue transfer. Anat Clin 1984;6:121–31.
3. Taylor GI, Palmer JH. The vascular territories (angiosomes) of the body: experimental study and clinical applications. Br J Plast Surg 1987;40:113–41.
4. Salmon M. Arteries of the skin. London: Churchill Livingstone; 1988.
5. Taylor GI, Caddy CM, Watterson PA, et al. The venous territories (venosomes) of the human body: experimental study and clinical implications. Plast Reconstr Surg 1990;86:185–213.
6. Morris SF, Taylor GI. Predicting the survival of experimental skin flaps with a knowledge of the vascular architecture. Plast Reconstr Surg 1993;92:1352–61.
7. Kroll SS, Rosenfield L. Perforator-based flaps for low posterior midline defects. Plast Reconstr Surg 1988; 81:561–6.
8. Koshima I, Soeda S. Inferior epigastric artery skin flaps without rectus abdominis muscle. Br J Plast Surg 1989;42:645–8.
9. Blondeel N, Vanderstraeten GG, Monstrey SJ, et al. The donor site morbidity of free DIEP flaps and free TRAM flaps for breast reconstruction. Br J Plast Surg 1997;50:322–30.
10. Blondeel PN. One hundred free DIEP flap breast reconstructions: a personal experience. Br J Plast Surg 1999;52:104–11.
11. Futter CM, Webster MH, Hagen S, et al. A retrospective comparison of abdominal muscle strength following breast reconstruction with a free TRAM or DIEP flap. Br J Plast Surg 2000;53:578–83.
12. Hamdi M, Weiler-Mithoff EM, Webster MH. Deep inferior epigastric perforator flap in breast reconstruction: experience with the first 50 flaps. Plast Reconstr Surg 1999;103:86–95.
13. Kroll SS, Sharma S, Koutz C, et al. Postoperative morphine requirements of free TRAM and DIEP flaps. Plast Reconstr Surg 2001;107:338–41.
14. Saint-Cyr M, Schaverien M, Arbique G, et al. Three- and four-dimensional computed tomographic angiography and venography for the investigation of the vascular anatomy and perfusion of perforator flaps. Plast Reconstr Surg 2008;121:772–80.
15. Schaverien M, Saint-Cyr M, Arbique G, et al. Arterial and venous anatomies of the deep inferior epigastric perforator and superficial inferior epigastric artery flaps. Plast Reconstr Surg 2008;121:1909–19.
16. Schaverien M, Saint-Cyr M, Arbique G, et al. Three- and four-dimensional arterial and venous anatomies of the thoracodorsal artery perforator flap. Plast Reconstr Surg 2008;121:1578–87.
17. Wong C, Saint-Cyr M, Arbique G, et al. Three- and four-dimensional computed tomography angiographic studies of commonly used abdominal flaps in breast reconstruction. Plast Reconstr Surg 2009; 124:18–27.
18. Saint-Cyr M, Wong C, Schaverien M, et al. Perforasome theory: vascular anatomy and clinical implications. Plast Reconstr Surg 2010;124(5):1529–44.
19. Holmstrom H. The free abdominoplasty flap and its use in breast reconstruction. An experimental study and clinical case report. Scand J Plast Reconstr Surg 1979;13:423–7.
20. Hartrampf CR, Scheflan M, Black PW. Breast reconstruction with a transverse abdominal island flap. Plast Reconstr Surg 1982;69:216–25.
21. Mosahebi A, Disa JJ, Pusic AL, et al. The use of the extended anterolateral thigh flap for reconstruction of massive oncologic defects. Plast Reconstr Surg 2008;122:492–6.
22. Saint-Cyr M, Schaverien M, Wong C, et al. The extended anterolateral thigh flap: anatomical basis and clinical experience. Plast Reconstr Surg 2009; 123:1245–55.
23. Koshima I, Moriguchi T, Fukuda H, et al. Free, thinned, paraumbilical perforator-based flaps. J Reconstr Microsurg 1991;7:313–6.
24. Allen RJ, Treece P. Deep inferior epigastric perforator flap for breast reconstruction. Ann Plast Surg 1994;32:32–8.
25. Offman SL, Geddes CR, Tang M, et al. The vascular basis of perforator flaps based on the source arteries of the lateral lumbar region. Plast Reconstr Surg 2005;115:1651–9.
26. Moon HK, Taylor GI. The vascular anatomy of rectus abdominis musculocutaneous flaps based on the deep superior epigastric system. Plast Reconstr Surg 1988;82:815–32.
27. Lin ZH. Clinical application of a paraumbilical axial flap: report of 16 cases (in Chinese). Zhonghua Zheng Xing Shao Shang Wai Ke Za Zh 1989;5: 249–50, 315.
28. Itoh Y, Arai K. The deep inferior epigastric artery free skin flap: anatomic study and clinical application. Plast Reconstr Surg 1993;91:853–63 [discussion: 864].
29. Munhoz AM, Ishida LH, Sturtz GP, et al. Importance of lateral row perforator vessels in deep inferior

epigastric perforator flap harvesting. Plast Reconstr Surg 2004;113:517–24.

30. Holm C, Mayr M, Hofter E, et al. Perfusion zones of the DIEP flap revisited: a clinical study. Plast Reconstr Surg 2006;117:37–43.

31. Angrigiani C, Grilli D, Siebert J. Latissimus dorsi musculocutaneous flap without muscle. Plast Reconstr Surg 1995;96:1608–14.

32. Thomas BP, Geddes CR, Tang M, et al. The vascular basis of the thoracodorsal artery perforator flap. Plast Reconstr Surg 2005;116:818–22.

33. Fujino T, Harasina T, Aoyagi F. Reconstruction for aplasia of the breast and pectoral region by microvascular transfer of a free flap from the buttock. Plast Reconstr Surg 1975;56:178–81.

34. Le-Quang C. Secondary microsurgical reconstruction of the breast and free inferior gluteal flap. Ann Chir Plast Esthet 1992;37:723–41 [in French].

35. Koshima I, Moriguchi T, Soeda S, et al. The gluteal perforator-based flap for repair of sacral pressure sores. Plast Reconstr Surg 1993;91:678–83.

36. Allen RJ, Tucker C Jr. Superior gluteal artery perforator free flap for breast reconstruction. Plast Reconstr Surg 1995;95:1207–12.

37. Blondeel PN, Van Landuyt K, Hamdi M, et al. Soft tissue reconstruction with the superior gluteal artery perforator flap. Clin Plast Surg 2003;30:371–82.

38. Blondeel PN. The sensate free superior gluteal artery perforator (S-GAP) flap: a valuable alternative in autologous breast reconstruction. Br J Plast Surg 1999;52:185–93.

39. Guerra AB, Metzinger SE, Bidros RS, et al. Breast reconstruction with gluteal artery perforator (GAP) flaps: a critical analysis of 142 cases. Ann Plast Surg 2004;52:118–25.

40. Granzow JW, Levine JL, Chiu ES, et al. Breast reconstruction with gluteal artery perforator flaps. J Plast Reconstr Aesthet Surg 2006;59:614–21.

41. Kerrigan CL, Daniel RK. The intercostal flap: an anatomical and hemodynamic approach. Ann Plast Surg 1979;2:411–21.

42. Hamdi M, Van Landuyt K, Monstrey S, et al. Pedicled perforator flaps in breast reconstruction: a new concept. Br J Plast Surg 2004;57:531–9.

43. Hamdi M, Van Landuyt K, de Frene B, et al. The versatility of the inter-costal artery perforator (ICAP) flaps. J Plast Reconstr Aesthet Surg 2006;59:644–52.

44. de Weerd L, Elvenes OP, Strandenes E, et al. Autologous breast reconstruction with a free lumbar artery perforator flap. Br J Plast Surg 2003;56:180–3.

45. Kato H, Hasegawa M, Takada T, et al. The lumbar artery perforator based island flap: anatomical study and case reports. Br J Plast Surg 1999;52:541–6.

Acoustic Doppler Sonography, Color Duplex Ultrasound, and Laser Doppler Flowmetry as Tools for Successful Autologous Breast Reconstruction

Geoffrey G. Hallock, MD[a,b,*]

KEYWORDS

- Acoustic Doppler sonography • Color duplex ultrasound
- Laser Doppler flowmetry • Breast reconstruction

Predictable and reproducible success in the transfer of autogenous tissues from any donor site for breast reconstruction must begin in the preoperative planning stage. Milton challenged the dictums of his time in recognizing that the sine qua non for best ensuring viability of any flap depended on its "circulation."[1] The precise identification of direct or indirect perforators[2] nurturing the assortment of available cutaneous flaps for breast reconstruction for just this reason has assumed paramount importance, as proper flap design must ensure inclusion of that perforator. A giant step taken in that direction was by Taylor and colleagues,[3] who first used the still ubiquitous acoustic Doppler probe to identify "dominant" skin perforators, and then planned safe flaps of "unusual dimensions and directions," along an axis connecting those perforators. The Doppler effect so evoked remains tacitly understood from basic principles of physics. Named after the Austrian physicist Christian Doppler, who actually identified the concept in 1842, this phenomenon is the change in frequency of a wave for an observer moving relative to the source of the wave.[4] This key principle has become ingrained in plastic surgery routines, and has since been expanded to include other evolving technologies such as color duplex ultrasound and laser Doppler flowmetry.

ACOUSTIC DOPPLER SONOGRAPHY

The typical acoustic Doppler probe is virtually universally available in every operating room and at every nursing station (**Fig. 1**). This compact device is highly portable, simple to use, and usually easy to interpret.

Acoustic Doppler sonography emits sound waves that reflect on a moving object relative to a fixed observer, and has a distinct phase shift according to the Doppler effect.[5] In flaps, the red blood cells are basically the only moving objects that scatter the incident source. The frequency of the latter will be shifted by an amount proportional to the number and velocity of the moving red blood cells in the specific target region, which predominantly represents intravascular blood flow. This results in the familiar and characteristic audible pitch that we differentiate between arteries and veins.[6]

To increase the specificity for locating a skin perforator, which is necessary to ensure flap boundaries will be designed to include that perforator, Mun and Jeon[7] have suggested a "perforator compression test." Because perforators are thinner walled and more superficial than their source vessel, and their course is approximately perpendicular to the skin surface, "true" perforators will

---

Disclosures: The author has nothing to disclose.
[a] Division of Plastic Surgery, Sacred Heart Hospital and The Lehigh Valley Hospitals, Allentown, PA, USA
[b] St. Luke's Hospital, Bethlehem, PA, USA
* 1230 South Cedar Crest Boulevard, Suite 306, Allentown, PA 18103.
E-mail address: pbhallock@cs.com

Clin Plastic Surg 38 (2011) 203–211
doi:10.1016/j.cps.2011.03.001

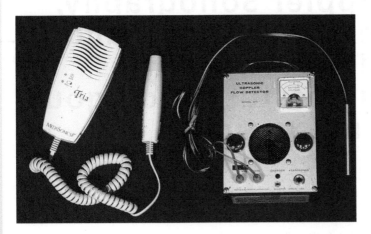

Fig. 1. Handheld acoustic Doppler ultrasound devices. Left, 5-MHz vascular probe (Medasonics, Newark, CA) used daily in our office practice; right, Ultrasonic Doppler Flow Detector with 8.9-MHz probe (Model 811-B, Parks Medical Electronics, Inc, Aloha, OR) native to our operating rooms and hospital floors.

be more easily compressed by an external force applied perpendicular to the skin surface. Thus, after finding a potential perforator with the audible Doppler probe, increased downward pressure will reduce and almost obliterate the original sound. Gradual release of the pressure will result in increasing loudness. Deeper or source vessels should have little change in sound intensity during such maneuvers.

As with any modality, there are limitations with acoustic Doppler sonography. The sensitivity may actually be too high (false positives), as often diminutive vessels inadequate to sustain a cutaneous flap can be found.[6] The specificity may be too low (false negatives), as vessels can be overlooked or missed because of background noise from larger vessels in the vicinity.[5] This latter characteristic also diminishes the capability of this device to allow accurate and consistent postoperative monitoring.

From a pragmatic standpoint, acoustic Doppler sonography has a short learning curve and will always be used by many, because it is readily available, as the sole technique for preoperative perforator identification,[8] or to corroborate the conclusions gleaned from other diagnostic modalities (**Fig. 2**). Because the probe can be sterilized, this is still the most practical means for intraoperative verification of perforators, as well as assessment of the location of recipient vessels.

COLOR DUPLEX ULTRASOUND

If a color spectrum is added to the moving component of conventional high-resolution, B-mode, gray-scale ultrasound, this combination of techniques is color duplex imaging.[9,10] The actual color observed on the monitor depends on the direction of flow in relation to the transducer used to perform the study. This can arbitrarily be assigned the color red or blue, with red usually chosen for the arteries and blue for the veins to simplify data interpretation, once each vessel type is identified correctly using the audible format included with most commercial machines.

Higher frequency transducers now permit scanning to superficial depths just below the skin level, with sensitivity to detect vessels with a diameter as small as 0.2 mm.[10,11] This so-called "power Doppler imaging"[11] is particularly relevant for investigations of perforators within the microcirculation, and was first used in plastic surgery for mapping of transverse rectus abdominis musculocutaneous (TRAM) flap perforators, usually then marked by coordinates centered about the umbilicus before breast reconstruction.[12,13] Fasciocutaneous perforators to deep inferior epigastric artery perforator (DIEAP) flaps, as well as other potential donor sites, have also been similarly localized.[6,9,14]

Depending on the orientation of the color duplex imaging transducer, the vessel orifice can be calibrated and peak systolic flow velocity determined from concomitant pulse-volume recordings; the take-off of perforators from the source vessel identified (**Fig. 3**); and the perforator intramuscular, subfascial, or epifascial course documented.[9,10,15]

Sensitivity in identifying perforators with color duplex imaging is high, but specificity is low, as only a small region can be examined at any time.[14,16] This equipment has limited availability, and usually a technician must be present to obtain consistent observations. Postoperative monitoring of buried DIEAP free flaps[15,17,18] has been reported, but the apparatus is just too awkward for routine continuous bedside or intraoperative monitoring (**Fig. 4**).

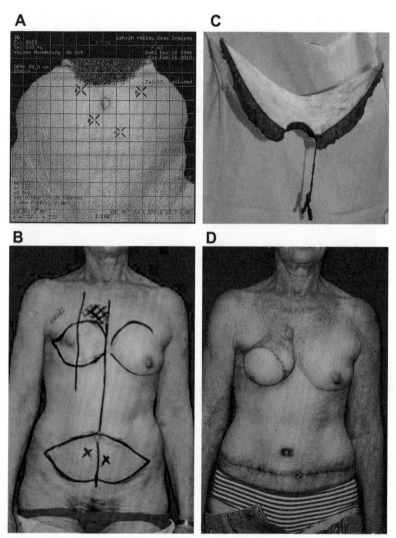

Fig. 2. (*A*) CTA study identified 4 dominant periumbilical perforators. (*B*) Acoustic Doppler ultrasound confirmed location of the 2 dominant infra-umbilical perforators, as marked by "x," within the preoperative outline of the desired flap. (*C*) DIEAP free flap based on CTA perforator #8. (*D*) Successful right breast autogenous tissue reconstruction with this DIEAP flap.

LASER DOPPLER FLOWMETRY

We have never attempted use of a scanning laser Doppler for preoperative regional perforator identification,[19] but have used surface laser Doppler flowmetry (LDF) for more than 20 years for both the intraoperative and postoperative monitoring of free flaps and sometimes pedicled flaps, following introduction of the concept by investigators from the Duke group.[20–22] More often than not, potential complications from pedicle kinking, an excessively tight closure, or anastomotic compromise are made apparent in the operating room even before clinical signs of flap embarrassment are obvious.[21] This noninvasive system provides an accurate,

objective display that is an almost ideal monitoring system (**Fig. 5**).

Laser Doppler flowmetry relies on tissue illumination by a coherent laser light, which has an emission wavelength of 780 nm from a 5-mW diode laser, as the reflecting source transmitted via a fiberoptic cable.[22] Although not visible to the naked eye, the Doppler shift of this reflected laser light can be calibrated via a computer within the monitor as a linear function of the average velocity of moving cells within the given flap.[23] Detection of blood flow and flow velocity up to an 8-mm depth is possible.[23] Real-time measurements of tissue perfusion are averaged over a predetermined time frame, and displayed either

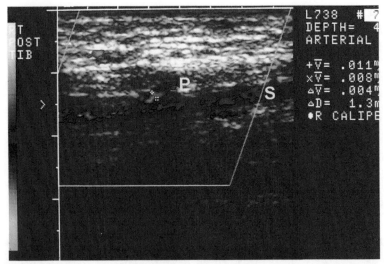

Fig. 3. Color duplex ultrasound scan, with color red distinguishing arteries. S, source vessel; P, perforator branch.

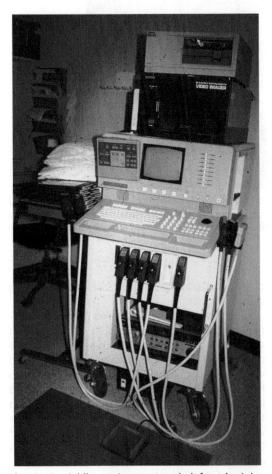

Fig. 4. Unwieldly equipment needed for obtaining color duplex ultrasound.

as a trend line (**Fig. 6**) or a number (see **Fig. 5**) that nursing personnel or even family members can watch for a significant variation, and does not require constant surveillance by a member of the surgical team.

Although each unit of measurement recorded corresponds to flow in mL/min/100 mg tissue,[20] absolute flow is not measured directly by this device, but rather provides a relative estimate that varies by patient and donor tissue.[20] Falsely elevated or positive flow values have been observed even under "no flow" conditions,[24] and can be caused by tissue vibrations, movement of the patient, or other artifacts.[21] Loss of arterial inflow typically results in an immediate and precipitous drop of flow values toward zero (see **Fig. 6**).[25–27] To provide a safety factor, we arbitrarily like to be notified if the display value drops below 1.0, which then mandates immediate clinical evaluation of the flap on our part. Venous obstruction is less obvious. A spiraling downward trend over time is consistent with an impediment of venous outflow (see **Fig. 6**).[23,25,26,28] This paradox of persistent positive flow values, albeit progressively smaller, can be explained, as some flow will continue into the flap up until the capacitance of the system is maximized.[22,26,29]

Intraoperative laser Doppler flowmetry has also allowed us to compare relative perfusion to zones of the abdomen (**Fig. 7**).[30] Poorly perfused regions should be discarded. Comparison of the relative perfusion from individual perforators, evaluated after alternating clamping, aids in deciding which

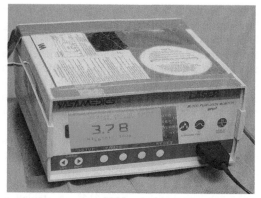

Fig. 5. Vasomedics Blood Perfusion Monitor (BMP²) (Vasamed, Inc, Eden Prairie, MN) used for flap monitoring. Note superimposed numeric display of relative flow value. Interconnect cable is plugged into machine at bottom right, and in turn transmits signal to a probe attached to the flap (as in **Fig. 7**).

perforators and their source vessels should be retained with the flap, which is especially valuable in deciding whether a superficial inferior epigastric artery flap is feasible in lieu of a deep inferior epigastric artery perforator flap. Probably the most critical time for assessing flap perfusion after completion of microanastomosis is during insetting. LDF surveillance during this period (see **Fig. 7**) helps to determine any pedicle compromise from kinking, stretching, or excessive pressure.

During normal monitoring, flow values will oscillate constantly, and so this should be expected. If the probe detaches from the flap, or anything obscures the interface between the flap and fiberoptic cable, such as a coagulum (**Fig. 8**), transmission of the laser signal will be blocked, and falsely low readings will be recorded.[21] On the monitor, a signal that the probe is "out of range"

may appear (see **Fig. 6**), and the last recorded value will no longer fluctuate, yet be permanently displayed, possibly leading to a false negative interpretation while the flap instead may be compromised.[31]

DISCUSSION
Basic Physics

The basic physics of the Doppler effect can be used to advantage as a tool for the planning and monitoring of any flap, including those used for autogenous breast reconstruction. Improved outcomes have paralleled technological advances in the ability to identify variations in the anatomic configuration of flaps, especially with regard to their intrinsic patterns of circulation. Acoustic Doppler sonography with the ubiquitous Doppler probe is still commonly used preoperatively to find skin perforators; however, admittedly it is limited, as operative findings can be completely different, such that sometimes specificity approaches 0%, the sound is muted as body mass increases, and the procedure will always be operator dependent.[32,33] Color duplex ultrasound also has a high sensitivity, and is an improvement on acoustic Doppler sonography in that perforator course and caliber can be visualized, and hemodynamic flow characteristics calculated.[6,34] However, obtaining this information is tedious even for an experienced technician, and is limited in its capacity to scan an entire body region.[6]

Multidetector Row CTA

Multidetector row computed tomographic angiography (CTA), as introduced by Masia and colleagues[35,36] for perforator flaps, has instead assumed priority in perforator identification. Comparison studies of imaging techniques by

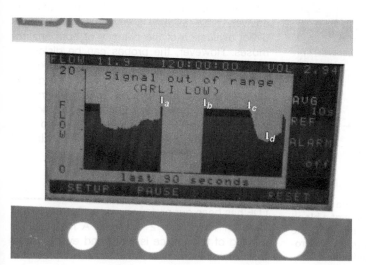

Fig. 6. Trend line of flow (ordinate) can also be displayed on BMP² monitor (Vasamed, Inc), here for a 90-second interval (abscissa). When arterial inflow was occluded (point "a"), a precipitous drop to almost zero flow was noted. When reestablished (point "b"), mean flow value reached a plateau about at the original level. Occlusion of venous outflow (point "c") resulted in gradual downward flow, followed by slow upward flow back to mean levels after occlusion was halted (point "d").

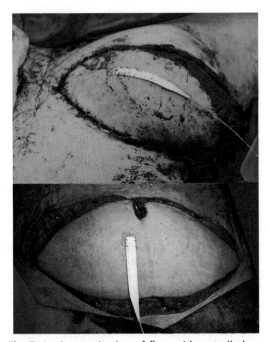

Fig. 7. In situ monitoring of flow with a sterile laser Doppler probe (Model 4409, Softflo Monitoring Probe, Vasamed, Inc) can differentiate perfusion to each zone of the abdominal flap (*bottom photograph*), or (*upper photograph*) intraoperative monitoring during insetting allows early recognition of a compromised flap.

Rozen and colleagues[37,38] and others[39] for DIEAP flaps for breast reconstruction have concluded that CTA is the new standard for preoperative perforator mapping,[37,38,40] as CTA had a 99.6% sensitivity for mapping perforators with a positive predictive value of 99.6%.[37,38] In addition, the

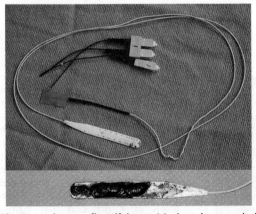

Fig. 8. Inadequate flow (false positive) can be recorded if probe is not in contact with flap because of a blood clot at the interface (*bottom photograph*), or if the fragile cable is broken (*upper photograph*, on microgrid), as here ripped apart by an agitated patient.

entire course of not just the source vessels and their branching patterns, including ascertaining the option of using the superficial inferior epigastric vessel, but also the perforators themselves and their trajectory within the muscle and toward the subdermal plexus, now allows the preoperative selection of the best alternative to capture maximal blood flow to the best available donor site (**Table 1**).

Yet, limitations of CTA beyond its expensive price tag must be considered. There may be a non-negligible lifetime risk of cancer from the unavoidable radiation exposure, which is additive for each successive scan.[41,42] A logistical problem not uncommon in our inner-city hospital is that all patients must be sent outside of network to get these sophisticated studies. Magnetic resonance angiography, again as shown by Rozen and colleagues,[43] may negate some of these concerns. Until MRI is commonly available and daily useful to then negate the need to use the acoustic Doppler. Acoustic Doppler sonography continues to have a role for the preoperative, intraoperative, and sometimes postoperative identification of perforators.[7] On the other hand, color duplex ultrasound has proven to be too cumbersome to be practical in this regard at the present.

Postoperative monitoring of any flap will always be essential, as salvage rates for compromised flaps are well known to be inversely proportional to the time interval between the onset of vascular insufficiency and clinical recognition.[22,24,44] The existence of numerous objective systems available to accomplish this implies that none is yet the ideal monitor.[23,28,45] Perhaps implantable 20-MHz ultrasonic probes, also relying on the Doppler principle, that are individually wrapped around both the arterial and venous pedicles will be the ultimate answer,[23,46,47] as their continuous signal allows direct evaluation of the patency of both anastomoses. However, the probes can be dislodged easily, unless part of the new GEM Flow Coupler (Synovis, Birmingham, AL) with integrated Doppler probe used for concomitant microanastomosis and monitoring. Also, this application is invasive, can be very expensive, and may never be readily available outside of specialized microsurgery centers.

Laser Doppler Flowmetry

LDF has been our preferred means for monitoring flaps for more than 2 decades. A major shortcoming of this device is that trend events rather than absolute numbers must be interpreted in

Table 1
Comparison of attributes of imaging systems

	Doppler Sonography	Color Duplex Imaging	Laser Doppler Flowmetry	CT Angiography
Perforator Localization:				
Sensitivity (true positive rate)	Good	Better	n/a	Best
Specificity (true negative rate)	Low	Low	n/a	Superior
Availability	Ubiquitous	Limited	Limited	Limited
Portability	Unlimited	Difficult	Somewhat	Difficult
Versatility (all operative phases)	No restriction	Limited	Monitoring	Restricted
Speed of Interpretation	Rapid	Tedious	Rapid	Moderate
Vessel Qualification:				
Caliber	Subjective	Accurate	n/a	Somewhat
Patency	Good	Excellent	n/a	Somewhat
Flow Characteristics	Subjective	Accurate	n/a	Marginal
Anomalies	Unrecognized	Good	n/a	Excellent
Pathology	Unrecognized	Good	n/a	Excellent
Establish hierarchy of perforator dominance	Subjective	Difficult	n/a	Excellent
Technical expertise	Minimal	Significant	Some	Considerable
Expense	Minimal	Not insignificant	Some	Considerable
Risk	None	Minimal	None	Radiation
Monitoring	Inexact	Difficult	Adequate	n/a

Abbreviation: n/a, not applicable.

nursing units by often-inexperienced personnel. More often than not, problems occur intraoperatively, especially with perforator flaps, and have been identified promptly by LDF to be then easily rectified to avoid the need for heroic postoperative salvage "take-backs." Actually, our major problem in using LDF is more pragmatic. This system has expensive start-up costs. Replacement interconnect cables and probes must come from a specific manufacturer. Regrettably, fiberoptic cables are easily crimped and broken, in spite of restraints imposed on agitated patients (see **Fig. 8**).

Basic Knowledge Still Required

In spite of ongoing technological advances even beyond this overview, the preoperative planning of any autogenous flap for breast reconstruction still requires a basic knowledge of the anatomy of each donor region, an anticipation of the general location of perforators,[48] and prediction of expected perfusion patterns.[49,50] Intraoperative and postoperative flap monitoring in some form will always be mandatory, as free flaps are always at risk for failure,[51] and salvage rates are reasonable when recognized early. The evaluation of flap color, turgor, temperature, and capillary refill, albeit subjective qualities, will always have a role.[23,28,44] Reliance on instrumental adjuncts alone can never completely eliminate the need for good clinical acumen.

SUMMARY

Successful autogenous tissue breast reconstruction requires retention of the best "circulation" to the chosen flap. Because intrinsic tissue movement in flaps primarily reflects intravascular blood flow, technology based on the Doppler effect can be apropos to detect or monitor such flow. Although CTA is currently the best imaging modality for identifying patterns of flap circulation, the old standby acoustic Doppler sonography is still useful to corroborate the location of perforators, and facilitate their intraoperative identification. The latter also remains a reasonable second-tier alternative if CTA is not available. Color duplex ultrasound is comparatively too tedious, time-consuming, and unwieldy to currently warrant continued use for this purpose. LDF is an objective monitoring system valuable for both intraoperative and postoperative monitoring of flap perfusion. Unfortunately, trends rather than absolute numbers must be interpreted by the monitoring team. When in doubt, clinical observation and subjective evaluation will always have an important role.

ACKNOWLEDGMENTS

David C. Rice, PE, Sacred Heart Hospital, Allentown, PA, and St Luke's Hospital, Bethlehem, PA, assisted with all microsurgery and Doppler studies.

REFERENCES

1. Milton SH. Pedicled skin-flaps: the fallacy of the length:width ratio. Br J Surg 1970;57:502–8.
2. Hallock GG. Direct and indirect perforator flaps: the history and the controversy. Plast Reconstr Surg 2003;111:855–66.
3. Taylor GI, Doyle M, McCarten G. The Doppler probe for planning flaps: anatomical study and clinical applications. Br J Plast Surg 1990;43:1–16.
4. Wikipedia. Doppler effect. Available at: http://en.wikipedia.org/wiki/Doppler_effect. Accessed July 4, 2011.
5. Hallock GG. Attributes and shortcomings of acoustic Doppler sonography in identifying perforators for flaps from the lower extremity. J Reconstr Microsurg 2009;25:377–81.
6. Hallock GG. Doppler sonography and color duplex imaging for planning a perforator flap. Clin Plast Surg 2003;30:347–57.
7. Mun GH, Jeon BJ. An efficient method to increase specificity of acoustic Doppler sonography for planning a perforator flap: perforator compression test. Plast Reconstr Surg 2006;118:296–7.
8. Knobloch K, Gohritz A, Reuss E, et al. Preoperative perforator imaging in reconstructive plastic surgery: current practice in Germany. Plast Reconstr Surg 2009;124:183e–4e.
9. Hallock GG. Color duplex imaging for identifying perforators prior to pretransfer expansion of fasciocutaneous free flaps. Ann Plast Surg 1994;32:595–601.
10. Hallock GG. Evaluation of fasciocutaneous perforators using color duplex imaging. Plast Reconstr Surg 1994;94:644–51.
11. Schwabegger AH, Bodner G, Rieger M, et al. Internal mammary vessels as a model for power Doppler imaging of recipient vessels in microsurgery. Plast Reconstr Surg 1999;104:1656–61.
12. Chang BW, Luethke R, Berg WA, et al. Two-dimensional color Doppler imaging for precision preoperative mapping and size determination of TRAM flap perforators. Plast Reconstr Surg 1994;93:197–200.
13. Rand RP, Cramer MM, Strandness ED. Color-flow duplex scanning in the preoperative assessment of TRAM flap perforators: a report of 32 consecutive patients. Plast Reconstr Surg 1994;93:453–9.
14. Blondeel P, Beyens G, Verhaeghe R, et al. Doppler flowmetry in the planning of perforator flaps. Br J Plast Surg 1998;51:202–9.
15. Numata T, Iida Y, Shiba K, et al. Usefulness of color Doppler sonography for assessing hemodynamics of free flaps for head and neck reconstruction. Ann Plast Surg 2002;48:607–12.
16. Miller JR, Potparic Z, Colen LB, et al. The accuracy of duplex ultrasonography in the planning of skin flaps in the lower extremity. Plast Reconstr Surg 1995;95:1221–7.
17. Yano K, Hosokawa K, Nakai K, et al. Monitoring by means of color Doppler sonography after buried free DIEP flap transfer [letter]. Plast Reconstr Surg 2003;112:1177.
18. Amerhauser A, Moelleken BR, Mathes SJ, et al. Color flow ultrasound for delineating microsurgical vessels: a clinical and experimental study. Ann Plast Surg 1993;30:193–203.
19. Komuro Y, Iwata H, Inoue M, et al. Versatility of scanning laser Doppler imaging to detect cutaneous perforators. Ann Plast Surg 2002;48:613–6.
20. Clinton MS, Sepka RS, Bristol D, et al. Establishment of normal ranges of laser Doppler blood flow in autologous tissue transplants. Plast Reconstr Surg 1991;87:299–309.
21. Heller L, Levin LS, Klitzman B. Laser Doppler flowmeter monitoring of free-tissue transfers: blood flow in normal and complicated cases. Plast Reconstr Surg 2001;107:1739–45.
22. Jenkins SD, Sepka RS, Barwick WJ, et al. Routine clinical use of laser Doppler flowmeter to monitor free tissue transfer: preliminary results. J Reconstr Microsurg 1987;3:281–3.
23. Smit JM, Zeebregts CJ, Acosta R, et al. Advancements in free flap monitoring in the last decade: a critical review. Plast Reconstr Surg 2010;125:177–85.
24. Marks NJ, Trachy RE, Cummings CW. Dynamic variations in blood flow as measured by laser Doppler velocimetry: a study in rat skin flaps. Plast Reconstr Surg 1984;73:804–10.
25. Hallock GG, Rice DC. A comparison of pulse oximetry and laser Doppler flowmetry in monitoring sequential vascular occlusion in a rabbit ear model. Can J Plast Surg 2003;11:11–4.
26. Yuen JC, Feng Z. Distinguishing laser Doppler flowmetric responses between arterial and venous obstructions in flaps. J Reconstr Microsurg 2000;16:629–35.
27. Hallock GG. Critical threshold for tissue viability as determined by laser Doppler flowmetry. Ann Plast Surg 1992;28:554–8.
28. Evans BC, Evans GR. Microvascular surgery. Plast Reconstr Surg 2007;119:18e–30e.
29. Yuen JC, Feng Z. Monitoring free flaps using the laser Doppler flowmeter: five-year experience. Plast Reconstr Surg 2000;105:55–61.
30. Hallock GG. Physiological studies using laser Doppler flowmetry to compare blood flow to the

zones of the free TRAM flap. Ann Plast Surg 2001; 47:229–33.

31. Hallock GG. A "true" false-negative misadventure in free flap monitoring using laser Doppler flowmetry. Plast Reconstr Surg 2002;110:1609–11.

32. Giunta RE, Geisweid A, Feller AM. The value of preoperative Doppler sonography for planning free perforator flaps. Plast Reconstr Surg 2000;105:2381–6.

33. Yu P, Youssef A. Efficacy of the handheld Doppler in preoperative identification of the cutaneous perforators in the anterolateral thigh flap. Plast Reconstr Surg 2006;118:928–33.

34. Tsukino A, Kurachi K, Inamiya T, et al. Preoperative color Doppler assessment in planning of anterolateral thigh flaps. Plast Reconstr Surg 2004;113:241–6.

35. Masiá J, Larrañaga J, Clavero JA, et al. The value of the multidetector row computed tomography for the preoperative planning of deep inferior epigastric artery perforator flap, our experience in 162 cases. Ann Plast Surg 2008;60:29–36.

36. Masia J, Clavero J, Larrañaga J, et al. Multidetector-row computed tomography in the planning of abdominal perforator flaps. J Plast Reconstr Aesthet Surg 2006;59:594–9.

37. Rozen WM, Phillips TJ, Ashton MW, et al. Preoperative imaging for DIEA perforator flaps: a comparative study of computed tomographic angiography and Doppler ultrasound. Plast Reconstr Surg 2008;121:9–16.

38. Rozen WM, Ashton MW, Stella DL, et al. The accuracy of computed tomographic angiography for mapping the perforators of the deep inferior epigastric artery: a blinded, prospective cohort study. Plast Reconstr Surg 2008;122:1003–9.

39. Scott JR, Liu D, Said H, et al. Computed tomographic angiography in planning abdomen-based microsurgical breast reconstruction: a comparison with color duplex ultrasound. Plast Reconstr Surg 2010;125:446–53.

40. Imai R, Matsumura H, Tanaka K, et al. Comparison of Doppler sonography and multidetector-row computed tomography in the imaging findings of the deep inferior epigastric perforator artery. Ann Plast Surg 2008;61:94–8.

41. Einstein AJ, Henzlova M, Rajagopalan S. Estimating risk of cancer associated with radiation exposure from 64-slice computed tomography coronary angiography. JAMA 2007;298(3):317–23.

42. Brenner DJ, Elliston CD. Estimated radiation risks potentially associated with full-body CT screening. Radiology 2004;232:735–8.

43. Rozen W, Stella D, Bowden J, et al. Advances in the preoperative planning of deep inferior epigastric artery perforator flaps: magnetic resonance angiography. Microsurgery 2009;29:119–23.

44. Chen KT, Mardini S, Chuang DC, et al. Timing of presentation of the first signs of vascular compromise dictates the salvage outcome of free flap transfers. Plast Reconstr Surg 2007;120:187–95.

45. Keller A. A new diagnostic algorithm for early prediction of vascular compromise in 208 microsurgical flaps using tissue oxygen saturation measurements. Ann Plast Surg 2009;62:538–43.

46. Oliver DW, Whitaker IS, Giele H, et al. The Cook-Swartz venous Doppler probe for the postoperative monitoring of free tissue transfers in the United Kingdom: a preliminary report. Br J Plast Surg 2005;58:366–70.

47. de la Torre J, Hedden W, Grant JH III, et al. Retrospective review of the internal Doppler probe for intra- and postoperative microvascular surveillance. J Reconstr Microsurg 2003;19:287–9.

48. Hallock GG. A primer of schematics to facilitate the design of the preferred muscle perforator flaps. Plast Reconstr Surg 2009;123:1107–15.

49. Rozen WM, Ashton MW, Le Roux CM, et al. The perforator angiosome: a new concept in the design of deep inferior epigastric artery perforator flaps for breast reconstruction. Microsurgery 2010;30:1–7.

50. Wong C, Saint-Cyr M, Mojallal A, et al. Perforasomes of the DIEP flap: vascular anatomy of the lateral versus medial row perforators and clinical implications. Plast Reconstr Surg 2010;125:772–82.

51. Khouri RK. Avoiding free flap failure. Clin Plast Surg 1992;19:773–81.

Maximizing the Use of the Handheld Doppler in Autologous Breast Reconstruction

Maurice Y. Nahabedian, MD*, Ketan M. Patel, MD

KEYWORDS

- Handheld Doppler • Autologous breast reconstruction
- Acoustic Doppler • Perforator flap breast reconstruction
- Flap monitoring

Over the past several decades, a variety of technological advancements have provided plastic surgeons with "tools" that have facilitated the ability to perform autologous reconstruction. The first tool was the acoustic Doppler ultrasound that was applied during the early years of flap reconstruction. Although surgeons had a general knowledge of the primary blood supply to a flap, little was known about the secondary vascularity, namely the perforators and other small vessels. The acoustic Doppler enabled surgeons to better understand the vascular anatomy relevant to a reconstructive procedure. Early studies were directed toward the donor sites to define perforator anatomy.[1,2] This information was useful for determining the cutaneous design and dimensions of a flap.

More recently, a number of technologically advanced devices have been introduced that have furthered our ability to define the vascular architecture. These include but are not limited to color duplex sonography, computerized tomographic angiography (CTA), magnetic resonance angiography (MRA), and fluorescent angiography.[2–8] Despite the benefits of these newer technologies, downsides related to cost, time, and interobserver variability have resulted in reluctance on the part of some surgeons to adopt these technologies. Instead, they have relied on classical techniques to define the vascular anatomy, such as the handheld acoustic Doppler. Although the acoustic Doppler does not provide the anatomic detail of these newer technologies, it still maintains a prominent role in soft tissue reconstruction and is very useful.

With the advent of perforator flap breast reconstruction, preoperative imaging and Doppler ultrasound technology has become increasingly important to better understand the vascular architecture. As a preoperative tool, the color duplex Doppler has been advocated.[9–11] Preoperative knowledge of the perforator anatomy can be important in the planning and design of flaps. The location and caliber of the perforators is variable for any given cutaneous surface. Benefits of Doppler sonography include real-time assessment, multiplanar capabilities, and evaluation of blood flow characteristics. The color duplex Doppler has been very effective in providing information regarding flow characteristics and directionality of flow.

The handheld acoustic Doppler is commonly used in the setting of autologous reconstruction. Like the color duplex Doppler, it can be used preoperatively but has the advantage of being used intraoperatively and postoperatively. It can be used as a sole modality or it can be used in conjunction with or to confirm the findings of CTA or MRA. This article focuses on the preoperative, intraoperative, and postoperative use of the handheld Doppler for free tissue transfer with an emphasis on perforator flap breast reconstruction.

Department of Plastic Surgery, Johns Hopkins University, Georgetown University Hospital, 3800 Reservoir Road NW, Washington, DC 20007, USA
* Corresponding author.
E-mail address: DrNahabedian@aol.com

Clin Plastic Surg 38 (2011) 213–218
doi:10.1016/j.cps.2011.03.006

DOPPLER PHYSICS

Human hearing can detect frequencies ranging from 20 Hz to 20 KHz. "Ultra"sound operates at frequencies higher (>20 KHz) than the audible range. Systems typically used in medicine have ranges far exceeding this, usually in the 1 to 20 MHz range. In the most basic state, ultrasound detection uses short pulses of high-frequency sound emitted into the body. Combinations of reflection, absorption, and scatter of sound waves to varying tissues are received to form the signal. With the addition of the Doppler effect to ultrasonography, the frequency of the reflected sound can be used to determine the direction of blood flow. Changes in signal intensity provide valuable information with regard to blood flow. Typically, the unidirectional Doppler ultrasound works by these principles.

DOPPLER: TRANSITIONING FROM PREOPERATIVE TO INTRAOPERATIVE TOOL

The handheld Doppler unit (**Fig. 1**) has proven to be one of the most versatile and widely used devices in autologous and especially microvascular breast reconstruction. Commonly used as a postoperative tool for free flap monitoring, preoperative and intraoperative efficacy have also been demonstrated.[12–15] Preoperatively, it is

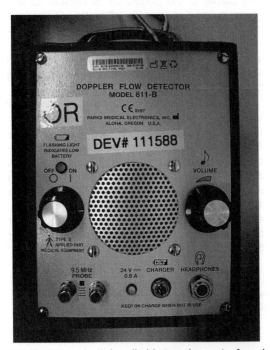

Fig. 1. A standard handheld Doppler unit found throughout nursing units and operating rooms.

sometimes used to localize perforator location on the cutaneous surface of the flap. Intraoperatively, it can be used to assist with perforator selection by discriminating between the various signal intensities. In the setting of abdominal or gluteal flap breast reconstruction, knowledge of perforator density and caliber can aid in faster and more effective flap elevation. Although some surgeons prefer the use of CTA, confirmation of the CTA data is almost always performed using a Doppler device. In a prior study using CTA for gluteal flap planning, it was demonstrated that there were an average of 11 perforators in the superior gluteal artery territory with a mean diameter of 0.6 mm. This was very similar to the comparative findings of Doppler ultrasound, as there were 9 perforators with a mean diameter of 0.4 mm.[16] The location of the CTA-documented perforators was confirmed using Doppler.[17]

The Doppler systems have played a prominent role in the planning and harvest of abdominal flaps. At the skin level, the handheld Doppler can predict the deeper location of abdominal perforators before any dissection. The periumbilical region consistently provides most usable abdominal perforators.[18] Giunta and colleagues[11] evaluated using the handheld Doppler in 46 patients before undergoing breast reconstruction. They found an average of 3.6 perforators in one-sided deep inferior epigastric perforator (DIEP) flap and 3.6 perforators in the superior gluteal artery perforator (SGAP) flap with preoperative Doppler assessment. Interestingly, when the preoperative Doppler skin signals were compared with intraoperative findings, a high false-positive rate of 47.6% and a false-negative rate of 11.0% were demonstrated. In addition, it was found that there was only minor discrepancy between the locations of the skin signal in relation to the deep location of each perforator (average of 0.8 cm vertically and 0.8 cm horizontally). This emphasizes the importance of possibly predicting the location of each perforator to approximately 1 square centimeter. The perforator compression test can potentially decrease a high false-positive rate. By applying external pressure with the Doppler probe, true perforator signals will vanish, leaving deeper source vessels as the remaining signal. This test can help to determine the origin of the Doppler signal.[19]

Clinical studies using Doppler ultrasound have been previously reported. Blondeel and colleagues[10] incorporated Doppler ultrasound in preoperative evaluation for patients who were to undergo DIEP and SGAP reconstruction. Approximately 4.5 perforators were indentified for each side of the abdominal flap and an average of 2.6

perforators for each SGAP flap. As related to the intraoperative findings, Blondeel and colleagues[10] reported a true positive rate of 80.6% and a positive predictive value of 91.9%. These studies highlight the sensitivity, sometimes oversensitivity, of the handheld Doppler at identifying cutaneous vessels. This is an important observation because many perforators are visualized during the elevation of an abdominal flap, many of which are small and will be sacrificed because of suboptimal location or caliber.

The success and efficiency of perforator-based breast reconstruction relies on the surgeon's experience with choosing the correct perforator(s) and with the technical aspect of perforator dissection. The handheld Doppler can aid the surgeon in selecting the best perforator(s) to optimize flow and perfusion within a flap and minimize the incidence of fat or partial flap necrosis. The following sections will describe the technique of using the handheld Doppler in identifying and selecting reliable perforators.

HANDHELD DOPPLER IN PERFORATOR SELECTION

The sequence of events for Doppler use is important. With the patient on the operating room table and before making any incisions, the handheld Doppler can be used to identify or reconfirm the location of perforators. In the case of an abdominal perforator flap, the perforator locations are marked with ink based on the acoustic Doppler signals (**Figs. 2** and **3**). It is important to appreciate the signal intensity and ensure that it is biphasic. Prior studies have demonstrated that most suitable perforators are located in the periumbilical region.[1,2,8] The number of perforators identified at

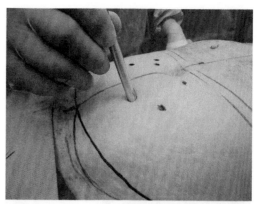

Fig. 3. Marking 3 to 4 strong intensity signals on each side is sufficient to begin the operation.

this stage is variable and will depend on the patient's body habitus and thickness of the adipocutaneous component of the abdominal wall. In general, however, approximately 3 to 4 perforators are marked.

During abdominal flap elevation, dissection usually proceeds in a lateral to medial direction, preserving all relevant perforator bundles encountered (**Fig. 4**). However, in a bilateral reconstruction, proceeding from medial to lateral is also advised. Throughout the dissection, a variety of perforators will be observed, some of which are small (<1 mm) and others larger (>1 mm). Smaller perforators without a palpable pulse lateral to the linea semilunaris are cauterized or clipped. Once the medial and lateral borders of the rectus abdominis are identified, the perforators are preserved and circumferentially dissected when possible. Typically, the goal is to select a perforator with a diameter of at least 1.5 mm; however, in some situations, a dominant perforator may not be evident and this may change the operative plan.

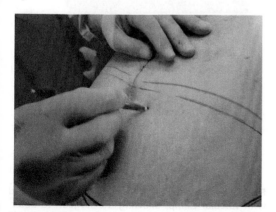

Fig. 2. Marking the location of perforators before surgery. Markings are made starting at the umbilicus and then moving away.

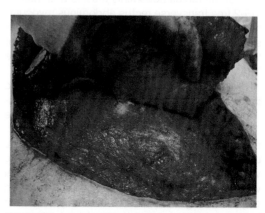

Fig. 4. After moving from lateral to medial, a series of perforator bundles are isolated.

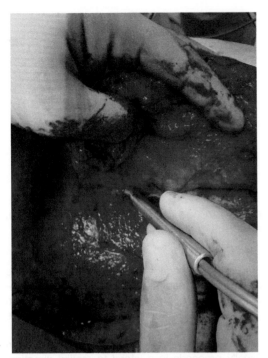

Fig. 5. A Doppler signal is obtained for each perforator and the intensity of each is compared.

The decisions as to whether a perforator flap or muscle-sparing flap will be performed are made at this juncture. The acoustic Doppler is especially useful at this time and can assist in making these decisions (**Fig. 5**). As the dissection proceeds along the anterior rectus sheath and larger dominant perforators are not visualized, an island of small perforators is created. Typically, the dimensions of this island range from 2 to 3 cm in width and 3 to 5 cm in length. The Doppler is used to confirm flow along the periphery of the fascial island. Typically, 3 to 5 small perforators are included. This island is usually within the middle third of the rectus abdominis muscle and thus an MS-2 free transverse rectus abdominus myocutaneous (TRAM) flap procedure is performed. Occasionally, the fascial island is along the medial or lateral segments of the muscle and an MS-1 free TRAM flap procedure is performed.

The method by which the probe is applied to the perforator(s) is important. It is directed perpendicular to each perforator being assessed. The probe is advanced along the length of the perforator, paying close attention to the signal quality. The presence of a biphasic arterial and monophasic venous signal are critical. Occasionally, a signal will be obtained that is monophasic or biphasic only. Selecting a perforator that is only venous or only arterial is obviously not advised when the goal is to perform a perforator flap.

Another important aspect of Doppler-related perforator selection is that perforators of different calibers will have different signal intensities. Some perforators will have a very robust signal and appear to be ideal, whereas others may have weak signal intensity. Generally speaking, larger perforators will be more robust, although small perforators can at times have very strong signal strength. It is important to assess signal strength and caliber when making decisions about perforator selection.

SEQUENTIAL CLAMPING TECHNIQUE

In situations where several usable perforators are isolated, the Doppler can be very useful in deciding which to select. The technique of selective occlusion of the perforator in conjunction with Doppler signals and flap characteristics has demonstrated benefit. After isolating usable perforators, vascular clamps can be placed on the perforators, leaving an isolated perforator to test for adequate flap perfusion (**Fig. 6**). The Doppler is applied to the remaining perforator to assess signal strength. It is also applied to the cutaneous surface to ensure that the location is appropriate. It is recommended to observe the flap for a few minutes to ensure that there are no color changes on the cutaneous surface. Color changes are interpreted as hyperemia, venous insufficiency, or arterial insufficiency. If arterial or venous insufficiency is evident, alternative perforators are selected. However, this may also be a sign that more than one perforator is necessary or that a muscle-sparing free TRAM flap may be indicated. Other factors that are important when making these decisions include the dimensions of the flap, the thickness of the flap, and the location of the

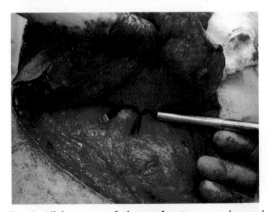

Fig. 6. All but one of the perforators are clamped with vascular clamps allowing the surgeon to determine if the perforator will support the entire flap. This test is coupled with evaluation of the skin paddle to determine if perfusion is adequate.

perforator relative to the flap dimensions. Once the flap has been harvested and the primary vascular pedicle has been defined, it is useful to use the acoustic Doppler along the length of the inferior epigastric and perforator vessels to ensure good flow based on the signal intensity and quality.

In addition to the utility of the handheld Doppler for the planning and execution of abdominally based flaps, it has been very useful for gluteal perforator flaps. Gluteal flaps differ from abdominal flaps in many ways but most notably in the perforator characteristics. Gluteal perforators are usually smaller and shorter than their abdominal counterparts. Thus, preoperative localization is critical to optimize one's success.

With the patient in the prone position, the handheld Doppler is used to identify the location of the perforators in the buttocks. This is an important preoperative maneuver because the delineation of the flap will depend on perforator location. In contrast to abdominal flaps, where it is desirable to have the perforator centrally located, with gluteal flaps, it is desirable to select a perforator that is peripherally located. The reasons for this relate to short length of the perforator and the technical advantage this confers when positioning the flap on the chest wall in preparation for the microvascular anastomosis. Although perforators are located on the medial and lateral buttock, the selection of a lateral perforator is preferred to provide slightly more perforator length. During the elevation of the flap, the Doppler is used much like previously described. Because of the tremendous branching patterns associated with the gluteal vessels, the combination of sequential clamping of branch points and Doppler ultrasound can facilitate selecting a perforator that will provide optimal length and caliber.

TIPS FOR POSTOPERATIVE MONITORING

Bedside clinical monitoring following flap reconstruction has proven successful for most reconstructive surgeons. False-positive take-back rates following standard monitoring are low. Despite this, newer, more innovative monitoring tools using microdialysis,[20] laser Doppler,[21] near-infrared spectroscopy,[22,23] and possibly glucose monitoring[24] have been developed to improve outcomes following flap reconstruction. Most of these newer technologies are expensive and there is a learning curve associated with use, leading most surgeons to rely on the handheld Doppler and clinical examination for postoperative monitoring.

When used for monitoring flaps postoperatively, it is important for all ancillary staff to appreciate the arterial and venous signal. Common practice is to delineate the precise location of this signal in the operating room and mark it with a superficial suture. It is important to realize that following a microvascular anastomosis it usually requires 45 to 60 minutes for the flap to equilibrate in terms of perfusion. Thus, a strong Doppler signal may not be evident initially on the cutaneous surface. Figus and colleagues[25] found statistically significant increases in flow within 1 hour after transfer. When on the monitoring unit, the nursing staff members are able to use this landmark for frequent flap evaluations. It is important to combine the ultrasound findings with clinical examination evaluating flap color, capillary refill, temperature, and turgor. In addition, venous augmentation maneuvers can be used to ensure adequate flap drainage. This is easily appreciated using the handheld Doppler by pressing on the flap at a point remote from the Doppler signal.

Implantable acoustic Doppler devices have gained popularity in free-flap reconstruction, especially head and neck reconstruction where buried free flaps are common.[26,27] In the setting of microvascular breast reconstruction, an implantable Doppler has been used by placing a fiberlike Doppler probe along the vascular anastomosis. This is a useful adjunct, especially in the patient following nipple-sparing mastectomy where there may be no cutaneous portion of the flap to visually monitor. These probes can be heard continuously or intermittently based on the degree of suspicion. Once the critical period of flap monitoring is complete, the probe is pulled out or cut at the level of the skin.

SUMMARY

The handheld Doppler has been classically used in all aspects of flap reconstruction. Although studies have shown that the Doppler may not provide the same anatomic detail as the other newer modalities such as CTA and MRA, the handheld Doppler remains a very useful and important tool for autologous reconstruction. In the preoperative setting, color duplex Doppler sonography is useful for identifying perforator location and caliber. Intraoperatively, the handheld Doppler is useful for assessing flow characteristics of the various perforators and to assist in selecting the most dominant or ideal perforator for a desired cutaneous territory. In the postoperative setting, the handheld Doppler is an excellent adjunct to the clinical examination and can reliably evaluate flap perfusion following reconstruction. When used thoughtfully and diligently, the handheld Doppler can be all that is needed to accurately and safely perform breast reconstruction.

REFERENCES

1. Rand RP, Cramer MM, Strandness DE Jr. Color-flow duplex scanning in the preoperative assessment of TRAM flap perforators: a report of 32 consecutive patients. Plast Reconstr Surg 1994; 93(3):453–9.
2. Chang BW, Luethke R, Berg WA, et al. Two-dimensional color Doppler imaging for precision preoperative mapping and size determination of TRAM flap perforators. Plast Reconstr Surg 1994;93(1): 197–200.
3. Hallock GG. Doppler sonography and color duplex imaging for planning a perforator flap. Clin Plast Surg 2003;30(3):347–57, v–vi.
4. Isken T, Alagoz MS, Onyedi M, et al. Preoperative color Doppler assessment in planning of gluteal perforator flaps. Ann Plast Surg 2009;62(2):158–63.
5. Rozen WM, Phillips TJ, Ashton MW, et al. Preoperative imaging for DIEA perforator flaps: a comparative study of computed tomographic angiography and Doppler ultrasound. Plast Reconstr Surg 2008; 121(1):9–16.
6. Rozen WM, Stella DL, Bowden J, et al. Advances in the pre-operative planning of deep inferior epigastric artery perforator flaps: magnetic resonance angiography. Microsurgery 2009;29(2):119–23.
7. Rozen WM, Stella DL, Phillips TJ, et al. Magnetic resonance angiography in the preoperative planning of DIEA perforator flaps. Plast Reconstr Surg 2008;122(6):222e–3e.
8. Scott JR, Liu D, Said H, et al. Computed tomographic angiography in planning abdomen-based microsurgical breast reconstruction: a comparison with color duplex ultrasound. Plast Reconstr Surg 2010;125(2):446–53.
9. Taylor GI, Doyle M, McCarten G. The Doppler probe for planning flaps: anatomical study and clinical applications. Br J Plast Surg 1990;43(1):1–16.
10. Blondeel PN, Beyens G, Verhaeghe R, et al. Doppler flowmetry in the planning of perforator flaps. Br J Plast Surg 1998;51(3):202–9.
11. Giunta RE, Geisweid A, Feller AM. The value of preoperative Doppler sonography for planning free perforator flaps. Plast Reconstr Surg 2000;105(7): 2381–6.
12. Disa JJ, Cordeiro PG, Hidalgo DA. Efficacy of conventional monitoring techniques in free tissue transfer: an 11-year experience in 750 consecutive cases. Plast Reconstr Surg 1999;104(1):97–101.
13. Solomon GA, Yaremchuk MJ, Manson PN. Doppler ultrasound surface monitoring of both arterial and venous flow in clinical free tissue transfers. J Reconstr Microsurg 1986;3(1):39–41.
14. Salgado CJ, Moran SL, Mardini S. Flap monitoring and patient management. Plast Reconstr Surg 2009;124(Suppl 6):e295–302.
15. Chubb D, Rozen WM, Whitaker IS, et al. The efficacy of clinical assessment in the postoperative monitoring of free flaps: a review of 1140 consecutive cases. Plast Reconstr Surg 2010;125(4):1157–66.
16. Rozen WM, Ting JW, Grinsell D, et al. Superior and inferior gluteal artery perforators: in-vivo anatomical study and planning for breast reconstruction. J Plast Reconstr Aesthet Surg 2011;64(2):217–25.
17. DellaCroce FJ, Sullivan SK. Application and refinement of the superior gluteal artery perforator free flap for bilateral simultaneous breast reconstruction. Plast Reconstr Surg 2005;116(1):97–103 [discussion: 104–5].
18. Liu LG. Color-flow duplex Doppler scanning study in the tram flap perforators: a report of 94 consecutive patients. Zhongguo Xiu Fu Chong Jian Wai Ke Za Zhi 2000;14(4):213–6 [in Chinese].
19. Mun GH, Jeon BJ. An efficient method to increase specificity of acoustic Doppler sonography for planning a perforator flap: perforator compression test. Plast Reconstr Surg 2006;118(1):296–7.
20. Udesen A, Lontoft E, Kristensen SR. Monitoring of free TRAM flaps with microdialysis. J Reconstr Microsurg 2000;16(2):101–6.
21. Yuen JC, Feng Z. Monitoring free flaps using the laser Doppler flowmeter: five-year experience. Plast Reconstr Surg 2000;105(1):55–61.
22. Repez A, Oroszy D, Arnez ZM. Continuous postoperative monitoring of cutaneous free flaps using near infrared spectroscopy. J Plast Reconstr Aesthet Surg 2008;61(1):71–7.
23. Colwell AS, Wright L, Karanas Y. Near-infrared spectroscopy measures tissue oxygenation in free flaps for breast reconstruction. Plast Reconstr Surg 2008;121(5):344e–5e.
24. Sitzman TJ, Hanson SE, King TW, et al. Detection of flap venous and arterial occlusion using interstitial glucose monitoring in a rodent model. Plast Reconstr Surg 2010;126(1):71–9.
25. Figus A, Ramakrishnan V, Rubino C. Hemodynamic changes in the microcirculation of DIEP flaps. Ann Plast Surg 2008;60(6):644–8.
26. de la Torre J, Hedden W, Grant JH 3rd, et al. Retrospective review of the internal Doppler probe for intra- and postoperative microvascular surveillance. J Reconstr Microsurg 2003;19(5):287–90.
27. Guillemaud JP, Seikaly H, Cote D, et al. The implantable Cook-Swartz Doppler probe for postoperative monitoring in head and neck free flap reconstruction. Arch Otolaryngol Head Neck Surg 2008;134(7):729–34.

Computerized Tomographic and Magnetic Resonance Angiography for Perforator-Based Free Flaps: Technical Considerations

Justin S. Lee, MD[a], Ketan M. Patel, MD[b], Zhitong Zou, MD[c], Martin R. Prince, MD, PhD[c], Emil I. Cohen, MD[a,*]

KEYWORDS
- Computed tomographic angiography
- Magnetic resonance angiography
- Preoperative planning • Surgical flaps

The advent of multidetector computed tomography (MDCT), with an ever-increasing number of detectors and faster gantry rotations, has revolutionized diagnostic radiology, allowing for rapid imaging at an increased resolution.[1] Coupling MDCT technology with improvements to intravenous contrast has made it possible to perform precise imaging during the arterial phase of contrast infusion increasing resolution of smaller vessels.[2] Computed tomographic angiography (CTA) is now routinely used in vascular, abdominal, and transplant surgery for its ability to provide accurate vascular anatomic detail. In most settings it has supplanted conventional invasive catheter angiography as the diagnostic imaging modality of choice for imaging blood vessels. CTA is a noninvasive method for preoperative planning, such as determining tumor resectability, arterial anatomy before organ donation, and

extent of peripheral vascular disease.[3–5] As advanced CTA has become mainstream, it is not surprising that new and novel applications have been developed in other specialties, including reconstructive surgery.

Over the last several decades, the use of perforator-based free flaps has gained appeal because of the reduction in donor-site morbidity common with conventional musculocutaneous flaps.[6,7] Successful perforator-based free flaps rely on selection of the appropriate dominant vessel supplying the vascular territory of the flap. Generally, anatomic variability increases in distal branches beyond the parent vessel. In addition, anatomic variability tends to increase as vessel size decreases. Improvements to surgical technique, allowing for the harvest of smaller, distal vascular segments has made knowledge of the native vascular anatomy critical during surgical

[a] Division of Vascular and Interventional Radiology, Department of Radiology, Georgetown University Hospital, 3800 Reservoir Road NW, Washington, DC 20007, USA
[b] Department of Plastic Surgery, Johns Hopkins University, Georgetown University Hospital, Washington, DC, USA
[c] Department of Radiology, Weill Cornell Imaging at New York Presbyterian Hospital, Weil Cornell and Columbia University, 416 East 55th Street, New York, NY 10022, USA
* Corresponding author.
E-mail address: Emil.I.Cohen@gunet.georgetown.edu

Clin Plastic Surg 38 (2011) 219–228
doi:10.1016/j.cps.2011.03.002
0094-1298/11/$ – see front matter © 2011 Elsevier Inc. All rights reserved.

dissection. Anatomic course and perforator diameter are important determining factors for flap perfusion.[8] Furthermore, understanding the perforator distribution and blood supply of a flap can impact the operative time and perfusion of the flap, ultimately affecting the outcome.[9]

Doppler ultrasound is used extensively for free-flap operative planning. Duplex sonography adds the ability to assess the rate of flow in addition to the acoustic characteristics of a vessel.[10] Unfortunately, ultrasound of any form is limited by its subjective nature, time required to perform a quality evaluation, and ultimately its reproducibility. Digital subtraction angiography was at one time considered the gold standard for the identification and mapping of vessels. However, it is an invasive procedure, which always has the risk of complications, such as vessel dissection and access-site hemorrhage. Evaluation of small, perforator-sized vessels requires selective angiography, which increases the risk of vessel injury and still fails to accurately depict the course of the vessel of interest in the surrounding soft tissue.[11]

Magnetic resonance angiography (MRA) and CTA have the advantages of being noninvasive methods of imaging vascular anatomy with high spatial resolution and soft-tissue detail that is easily reproducible. MRA has the advantage of not using ionizing radiation, which is a consideration, particularly when dealing with younger patient populations. These two imaging modalities are discussed further as tools for preoperative evaluation in perforator-based flap reconstruction.

Alonso-Burgos and colleagues[12] published one of the first reports using CTA for reconstructive surgery in which 6 patients were evaluated using CT for deep inferior epigastric perforator (DIEP) tissue flap planning. A 4-detector row MDCT scanner was used with 150 mL of iodixanol contrast medium. The investigators obtained a slice thickness of 1.25 mm and reformatted images into multiplanar reformats, maximum intensity projections (MIP), and 3-dimensional (3-D) volume-rendered images. Arterial perforators were identified and evaluated for vessel diameter, fascial penetration pattern, intramuscular course, origin from the deep inferior epigastric artery, and other anatomic variations. In all 6 patients, accurate main perforators were identified on CTA with no additional vessels found at the time of the surgery. In addition, CTA provided important adjunctive preoperative information, such as muscular diastasis, abdominal wall hernia, and fatty infiltration of potential flaps. This early experience with an early 4-detector row scanner showed promising results for CTA as a noninvasive means for presurgical planning.

The same year Masia and colleagues[13] published a retrospective review of 66 DIEP flap reconstructions in which CTA was used for preoperative planning. The investigators found an average time saved of 1 hour and 40 minutes in cases with preoperative CTA. There were 2 cases with partial necrosis and 1 total failure in the group without prior CTA and only 1 partial necrosis case in the CTA group. The investigators thought that CTA offered a high sensitivity, specificity, and 100% positive predictive value. Furthermore, they were able to highlight the value of CTA as a tool to reduce operative time by identifying the most suitable perforator allowing safe ligation of other smaller vessels.

In 2008, Rozen and colleagues[14] published a series of articles using CTA for DIEP and superficial inferior epigastric artery (SIEA) flaps (**Table 1**). The first report included 75 patients using a 64-detector row scanner the images reconstructed as 1-mm slices. Of the 75 patients, they specifically describe seven cases in which CTA actually changed the operative plan due to the anatomy, particularly patients with prior abdominal wall surgical history. Later, a second study performed by the same group evaluated 104 reconstructions to determine if there were outcome differences after preoperative CTA.[15] The investigators concluded that preoperative CTA was associated with a statistically significant decrease in flap complications, donor-site morbidity and operative stress for the surgeon. In a similar study, Smit and colleagues[16] also demonstrated a trend toward the reduction in surgical time. Their study compared 70 patients who were evaluated preoperatively with CTA and 68 by preoperative Doppler ultrasound. There was a statistically significant decrease in surgical time and no flap complications in the CTA group.

Despite CTA strengths in arterial imaging, limitations do exist. A comparison study of Doppler to CTA for DIEP flap planning in 2010 evaluated 45 patients preoperatively examined with both Doppler and CTA. In this series, the dominant perforator used for the flap was found in 44 patients with Doppler and 41 patients with CTA.[17] Additionally, among CTA patients, there was a disagreement in perforator size described on the CTA compared with what was found during surgery. Overestimation on the CTA was attributed to a summation of the perforating artery and adjacent vein during measurement, likely secondary to volume averaging. The investigators did find that CTA provided a better analysis of the intramuscular course of the vessels as well as assessment of superficial venous communication, and that overall CTA provided a global picture to the surgeon.

MRA has continued to improve on its ability to visualize vessels distinctly within adjacent soft

Table 1
Comparison of recently available publications evaluating CTA for DIEP flap harvesting

Authors	Year	Number of Patients/Flaps	Free Flap	Reported Success Rate (%)
Alonso-Burgos et al[12]	2006	6	DIEP	100
Masia et al[13]	2006	66	DIEP	100
Rozen et al[14,15,a]	2008	75	DIEP/SIEA	100
Rozen et al[14,15]	2008	88	DIEP	100
Schaverien et al[27]	2008	12	DIEP	—
Rozen et al[14,15]	2008	10	DIEP	—
Phillips et al[21]	2008	65	DIEP/SIEA	—
Clavero et al[28]	2009	126	DIEP	100
Masia et al[29]	2009	162	DIEP	99
Rozen et al[30]	2009	26	DIEP	—
Smit et al[16]	2009	70	DIEP	100
Pacifico et al[31]	2009	60	DIEP	—
Rozen et al[b]	2009	6	DIEP	100
Whitaker et al[32]	2009	325	DIEP	—
Rozen et al[33]	2009	10	DIEP	100
Kim et al[34]	2010	58	ALT	—
Chen et al[35]	2010	32	ALT	83
Gattaura et al[36]	2010	100	DIEP	—
Masia et al[26]	2010	357	DIEP	100
Zhang et al[37]	2010	4	ALT	—
Visscher et al[38]	2010	10	DIEP	—
Katz et al[39,c]	2010	86	DIEP	—
Ting et al[40,a]	2010	1	DCIA	—
Rad et al[41,c]	2010	12	SGAP/LSGAP	—
Gacto-Sanchez et al[42,b]	2010	70	DIEP	10
Cina et al[17,b]	2010	45	DIEP	91
Ribuffo et al[43]	2010	41	OFFF	100

[a] Case reports.
[b] Connotes a comparison of Doppler ultrasound and CTA.
[c] Studies using CTA but not evaluating CTA outcome.
Abbreviations: ALT, anterolateral thigh flap; OFFF, osteocutaneous fibula free-flap; SGAP/LSGAP, superior gluteal artery perforator/lateral supragenicular artery.

tissue and lack of ionizing radiation. This ability is in large part because of faster gradients and improved sequences. A recent study confirmed the potential of MRA for preoperative planning.[18] Continued work in this area especially with newer technological advancements, including the introduction of blood-pool contrast agents, should ultimately give MRA a distinct advantage in this field.

CTA TECHNIQUE

Proper acquisition of the raw data is critical for correct vascular assessment of the donor area. Although CTA acquisition involves the manipulation of a small set of variables, familiarity with them insures correct image acquisition and therefore reduces the risk for repeated contrast boluses and exposures to ionizing radiation.

PATIENT PREPARATION

Enteric contrast is avoided before any CTA acquisition. Patients are asked to disrobe and only wear a hospital gown without tying it. Because 3-D shaded surface rendering will be used to depict anatomic location of the perforators in relation to the overlying skin, any material distorting the normal contour of the abdomen is avoided. Furthermore, patients are positioned with arms at their sides to again replicate the natural neutral position of the abdominal soft tissue during the future surgery. For similar reasons no retention devices are used.

A large-gauge (18 gauge or larger) peripheral intravenous line is placed in the antecubital region of the arm. The large size is required for the rapid infusion of contrast, which is essential for adequate opacification of small vessels. Such vessels, as in the case of abdominal perforators, which range in size between 1 to 4 mm, require an adequate contrast bolus to be properly imaged. Extensive literature regarding contrast bolus is available in the coronary CTA literature regarding the ideal rate of contrast infusion for vessels of similar size in that region of the body. As a general rule, approximately 1 to 2 g of iodine is injected per second to allow the best visualization of vessels of this caliber.[2,19,20] Although iodine concentrations per milliliter of contrast vary for CTA, the highest available concentration is used. This concentration is generally 350 to 370 mg/mL in the United States and 400 mg/mL in Europe. The principle can be simply stated: a lower iodine concentration will require a higher injection rate to obtain equivalent image quality. Furthermore, most contrast agents have a high viscosity and therefore generate high pressures at the suggested high flow rates. It is therefore prudent to place the largest intravenous access feasible and adjust the flow rate accordingly. In most patients flow rates between 4 to 6 mL/s should be attainable keeping in mind that patients with a larger body habitus will require higher flow rates. Finally, when performing examination with high injection rates it is recommended to use a test bolus of at least 10 mL of normal saline to test the intravenous access before infusion of contrast bolus. This practice will minimize the risk of infiltration of the iodinated contrast, which in turn may cause significant morbidity ranging from arm discomfort to a compartment syndrome.

CT EXAMINATION

Although a routine abdomen and pelvis CTA can provide adequate coverage, this would expose patients to unnecessary additional ionizing radiation. The area of interest is from the origin of the inferior epigastric artery to a level approximately 4 cm above the umbilicus. In the interest of lowering exposure to ionizing radiation, it is possible to obtain all the necessary information for preoperative planning by limiting the scan area to this region when acquiring the images. The study should be performed on a CT machine capable of rapid image acquisition at a high resolution. Generally, most machines on the market today, with the capability of 16 or greater

simultaneous slice acquisition, have the necessary specifications to perform a quality examination.

The examination may be performed in the traditional cranio-caudad mode after an aortic threshold of 100 Hounsfield units is reached or further optimized by placing the region of interest on the common femoral artery and scanning in a caudo-craniad fashion as has been described previously.[21] This later modification has been advocated for better timing of the examination for the arterial phase of the abdominal perforator vessels by taking advantage of the direction these vessels enhance.

The amount of contrast will vary depending on the speed of image acquisition. Thus, in a faster machine less contrast can be used. Empirically, 80 mL of contrast will suffice for most examinations because of the narrow area of interest and the possibility to complete most examinations in less than 10 seconds. However, calculation of the exact dose required may be obtained by the following formula:

Contrast volume (mL) = scan duration (delay to scan start from threshold trigger + scan time) X injection rate (typically 4–5 mL/s).

Note on Dose Modulation

Most scanners today modulate the x-ray beam energy (defined as milliampere-second) based on the topogram obtained at the beginning of the examination or a similar algorithm. Subjective reporting of blurring of the vessels of interest caused by this technique has led investigators to disable this option during image acquisition of DIEP flap CTA.[22]

MRA TECHNIQUE

Despite recent excitement about the potential of 3.0-T machines when compared with the standard 1.5-T MR imaging for various parts of the body,[23] for perforator flap MRA, characteristics other than signal-to-noise ratio take precedence. For instance, it is more important to have good suppression of the subcutaneous fat over a wide field of view to include all the abdominal subcutaneous fat and to minimize artifacts from adjacent air containing viscera. Accordingly, the scanner that has the best magnetic field homogeneity, shimming, and largest field of view is generally better; in most cases, this is a scanner with a 1.5-T field scanner.

Because imaging small perforators on MRA over a large field of view is capitalizing on MR technology, a newer state-of-the-art scanner with top gradient performance and a high-quality body or cardiac, 8- to 32-channel phased array coil are essential.[24]

PATIENT PREPARATION

Unlike CTA, fasting is not necessary before MRA because the gadolinium contrast rarely causes nausea/vomiting. However, high-protein foods can simulate contrast and therefore interfere with the postcontrast imaging essential for a quality examination. Accordingly, some have advocated a mild bowel preparation or avoidance of high-protein meals the day beforehand or even 0.5 mg glucagon intravenously to decrease peristalsis. A phase encoding gradient from right to left can also minimize these artifacts. The ideal gadolinium preparation, gadofosveset trisodium, sometimes causes transit pelvic tingling. Informing patients about this before the examination helps to avoid surprises that can cause motion during the arterial phase of contrast injection.

The umbilicus is used as a reference for locating the abdominal perforators. Its marking with a vitamin E capsule may be undertaken to aid in better localization before patient positioning in the MR gantry. Additional important landmarks may also be marked, such as the gluteal crease, pubic symphysis, and sternal notch.[25]

PATIENT POSITIONING IN SCANNER

Normally MRA scanning is performed in the supine position. However, positioning patients prone minimizes motion artifact in the anterior subcutaneous fat and abdominis rectus muscles especially if patients are not able to suspend breathing for the long MRA scan time with blood pool contrast agents, such as gadofosveset trisodium. In fact, eliminating the need for breath holding allows acquisition of high-resolution 512 × 512 matrix 3-D images over a 3- to 4-minute scan duration during the blood pool phase.

The umbilicus is a critical reference landmark for localizing each perforator in the anterior abdominal wall, it is therefore important to ensure its midline positioning before scanning patients. If need be, breast coils may be used in addition to the abdominal coils to image the breast tissue for possible volume analysis and graft size planning. After completing prone imaging, patients can be switched to supine position for a final 3-D acquisition of medial thigh perforators, if necessary.

PULSE SEQUENCES

As with all MRA, single-shot T2 sequences may be obtained initially to aid in better localization of the area of interest as well as further characterization of any abnormalities. The primary sequence for visualizing the perforators is a 3-D spoiled gradient echo sequence with separation of fat and water

signals. Ideally this is a multi-echo sequence reconstructed with 2-point or 3-point Dixon methodology. If the latter is not available, traditional fat suppression or subtraction imaging can be used. But no matter what technique is used ultimately, a noncontrast series must be obtained to ensure that the fat suppression is working properly in the areas of interest. Any drift of the fat suppression onto the water peak in the area of interest should be corrected because this will cause obscuration of the vessels of interest. Techniques used to minimize poor fat saturation include a reduced field of view, shimming, or adjusting the center frequency.

Typically, slices are 3 mm thick with 2-fold zero padding for a 1.5-mm spacing and 1.5-mm overlap of reconstructed images. Timing of the gadofosveset trisodium bolus to the arterial phase can be done with fluoroscopic triggering. Gadofosveset trisodium can be hand injected at about 1 mL/s. The arteries and veins generally run in pairs and are better visualized on a higher resolution, 512 × 512 matrix equilibrium blood pool phase axial image that typically is acquired over 3 to 4 minutes without using the parallel acquisition technique. The latter is often used to shorten acquisition times at the expense of signal intensity. Near the end of the examination, delayed imaging in sagittal and coronal planes, at a lower resolution, with activation of 2-fold parallel imaging and breath holding is obtained to provide an overview of the anatomy.[26]

IMAGE RECONSTRUCTION

As with any CTA/MRA evaluation, most of the relevant information can be ascertained from the

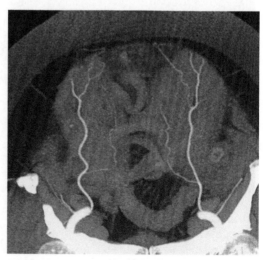

Fig. 1. Coronal MIP image from a CTA showing the patency of the inferior epigastric system on a patient being evaluated for a DIEP flap reconstruction. This image plane can aid in differentiating the branching patterns.

source images where a general impression of the vascular anatomy of the donor site is obtained. Subsequently, axial and coronal MIP images (**Fig. 1**) are compiled to confirm the anatomy and to generate images for the operating surgeon. This later set of images is often supplemented by volume-rendered 3-D images demonstrating the anatomic relationship of the vessels of interest with body landmarks, such as skin and the umbilicus (**Fig. 2**). Many workstations also have the capability of overlapping a grid on the obtained images to allow the surgeon to accurately calculate the course of the donor blood vessel relative to landmarks, such as the umbilicus.

Various color schemes can be used to denote the vessel of interest, muscle, and facial planes to facilitate surgical planning. The points that must be addressed are the course and branching of the arteries, locations of perforators, and obvious venous anomalies. Of the 3, the course of the artery is most important and special note must be made of any long intramuscular course. The diameter of the inferior epigastric artery and perforators must also be noted, specifically if it is felt that the vessels are of small caliber (<1 mm).

When reviewing MIP images, a slab that is 8 to 20 mm in thickness is used in multiple oblique planes. Most workstations allow placement of

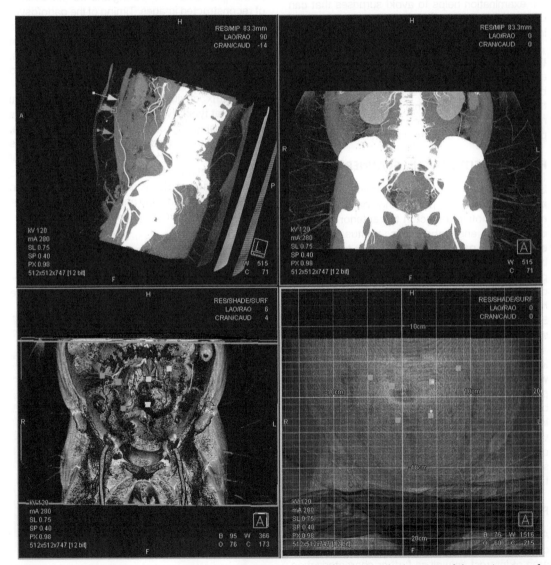

Fig. 2. Composite CTA image represents 3-D shaded surface image illustrating the location of the patient's perforators in relation to the umbilicus. Similarly, the coronal image shows the course and size of the vessels of interest without the adjacent soft-tissue structures. Composite images can allow more accurate localization of each perforator of interest.

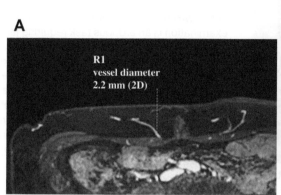
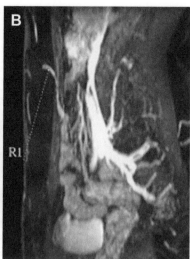

Fig. 3. A right abdominal perforator R1 (vessel diameter 2.2 mm) coming through the right rectus muscle on (A) axial and (B) sagittal maximum-intensity projection images from an MRA examination.

arrows or other such annotations in a selected plane and transfer them to other orthogonal planes to mark the course of a selected vessel (see **Fig. 2**).

In MRA evaluation, high-resolution 3-D blood pool phase images give the best delineation of perforating vessels. For each perforator, intramuscular course can be depicted on a thin slab MIP, which combines several slices to show the perforator over a longer path. The diameter and distance between the marker and perforators also need to be recorded (**Figs. 3–6**).

COMPARISON OF TECHNIQUES

When comparing duplex ultrasound, CT angiography, and MR angiography there are benefits and drawbacks of each technique. These strengths and weaknesses are related to the spatial and contrast resolution of each respective modality. Ultrasound is ideally suited to assess superficial structures in great detail because of its high spatial resolution of superficial structures and the ability to map vessels by using duplex examination. The limitations of ultrasound are caused by its low contrast resolution, which manifests as operator dependence and interobserver variability of the technique. Furthermore, patient attributes can affect the examination. For example, body habitus of an obese patient can limit evaluation as the spatial resolution of ultrasound is significantly diminished by object depth. This in turn may result in under description of the number of vessels present in the area of interest. A further limitation is the inability of the technique to generate information relating to the 3-D course of the vessels is an additional limitation. Ultrasound does have the advantage of the lowest total cost of the group.

CTA acquisitions are rapid and thorough with little dependence on the operator. It has the highest

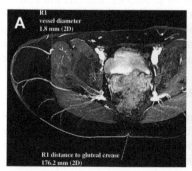
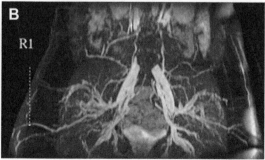

Fig. 4. A right gluteal perforator R1 (vessel diameter 1.8 mm) on (A) axial and (B) coronal MIP images from an MRA examination. On Figure 4A, the distance from the gluteal crease to R1 perforating the gluteus medius was measured as 176.2 mm.

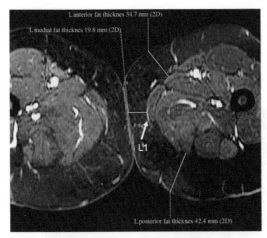

Fig. 5. A left gracilis muscle perforator L1 on MRA was shown on Fig. 5. The fat thickness from the inner surface of adductor longus muscle, L1 perforation and adductor magnus muscle to the inner skin border was measured 34.7, 19.8 and 42.4 mm separately.

spatial resolution, although it ranks behind MRA for contrast resolution. Given the inherent density differences between vessels, muscle and fat along with the small caliber of the vessels of interest, CTA can easily visualize the vessels of interest. The main drawbacks of CTA are ionizing radiation and the need for intravenous contrast, limiting its use in patients with marginal renal function. Current dose reduction algorithms in use significantly reduce but do not eliminate this weakness.

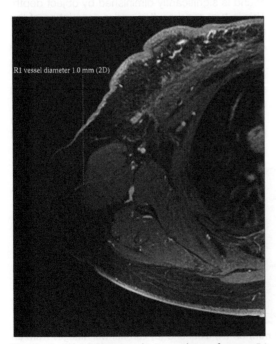

Fig. 6. A right latissimus dosi muscle perforator R1 (vessel diameter 1.0 mm) from an MRA examination.

MRA has the highest contrast resolution but the lowest spatial resolution and highest overall cost. The availability of high-quality MR machines with adequate technical specifications to allow for high-resolution MRA imaging is not uniform. Delineating which machines are adequate to perform an examination is an arduous task requiring familiarity with details about the individual machines. Almost all CT scanners possessing 16 or greater detector rows are adequate for noncardiac CTA, the same cannot be said of all 1.5-T scanners prevalent in the clinical practice. Factors vital to obtaining high-resolution MRA images, such as the gradient type, are not readily available. Furthermore, MR examinations are more arduous for patients because of their scan durations.

MRA does have the advantage of using magnetic fields rather than ionizing radiation, which has little known deleterious effects and holds great promise for vascular imaging given its unparalleled contrast resolution. Research in to image quality, vessel sharpness, and number of perforators visualized has shown great promise for gadofosveset trisodium compared with traditional extracellular contrast agents, such as gadobenate dimeglumine. Future MRA imaging will focus on improving image quality; using techniques, such as homogeneous fat suppression; diminishing bright bowel signal on the anterior abdominal wall; and using blood pool contrast agents to acquire a sharper edge of the perforator flap. As with CTA, the cost of the examinations may be justified by the time saved during the actual harvesting procedure by having a clear vascular map before the procedure.

Studies comparing vessel diameter measured on CTA, MRA, and ultrasound have repeatedly shown that size estimations based on cross-sectional imaging (CTA/MRA) is less accurate than on ultrasound.[17] This finding is not surprising because the spatial resolution of an ultrasound examination is much higher when dealing with superficial structures, such as the inferior epigastric arteries and their perforators. Nevertheless, in clinical practice it is often adequate to simply differentiate vessels, which are of less than adequate diameter for the pending procedure.

SUMMARY

Perforator-based free flaps, such as the DIEP flap, have become the standard approach for reconstructive surgery. As the volume of reconstruction increases, the need for a quick, reliable, and reproducible method for preoperative evaluation is necessary. Adequate evaluation of the vascular supply of free flaps is critical to the success of the operation. MDCT technology currently provides the ability to perform accurate imaging of vascular anatomy, improving preoperative information. The result is diminished operative time and improved outcomes. The limitations of CTA regarding intravenous contrast and spatial resolution compared with Doppler ultrasound suggest that the technologies need to be applied based on patient and surgeon needs. MRA technology may eliminate some of the deleterious effects of CTA while maintaining superior imaging quality needed for reconstruction planning. Radiation exposure is controversial, implying at best that the overall benefit of the study needs to be weighted against the individual need of each case.

REFERENCES

1. Rubin GD, Walker PJ, Dake MD, et al. Three-dimensional spiral computed tomographic angiography: an alternative imaging modality for the abdominal aorta and its branches. J Vasc Surg 1993;18:656–64 [discussion: 665].

2. Kim DJ, Kim TH, Kim SJ, et al. Saline flush effect for enhancement of aorta and coronary arteries at multidetector CT coronary angiography. Radiology 2008; 246:110–5.

3. Foley WD, Stonely T. CT angiography of the lower extremities. Radiol Clin North Am 2010; 48:367–96, ix.

4. Vrtiska TJ, Fletcher JG, McCollough CH. State-of-the-art imaging with 64-channel multidetector CT angiography. Perspect Vasc Surg Endovasc Ther 2005;17:3–8.

5. Winston CB, Lee NA, Jarnagin WR, et al. CT angiography for delineation of celiac and superior mesenteric artery variants in patients undergoing hepatobiliary and pancreatic surgery. AJR Am J Roentgenol 2007;189:W13–9.

6. Nahabedian MY, Tsangaris T, Momen B. Breast reconstruction with the DIEP flap or the muscle-sparing (MS-2) free TRAM flap: is there a difference? Plast Reconstr Surg 2005;115:436–44 [discussion: 445–6].

7. Man LX, Selber JC, Serletti JM. Abdominal wall following free TRAM or DIEP flap reconstruction: a meta-analysis and critical review. Plast Reconstr Surg 2009;124:752–64.

8. Patel SA, Keller A. A theoretical model describing arterial flow in the DIEP flap related to number and size of perforator vessels. J Plast Reconstr Aesthet Surg 2008;61:1316–20 [discussion: 1320].

9. Rozen WM, Ashton MW. Improving outcomes in autologous breast reconstruction. Aesthetic Plast Surg 2009;33:327–35.

10. Giunta RE, Geisweid A, Feller AM. The value of preoperative Doppler sonography for planning free perforator flaps. Plast Reconstr Surg 2000;105: 2381–6.

11. Lell M, Tomandl BF, Anders K, et al. Computed tomography angiography versus digital subtraction angiography in vascular mapping for planning of microsurgical reconstruction of the mandible. Eur Radiol 2005;15:1514–20.

12. Alonso-Burgos A, García-Tutor E, Bastarrika G, et al. Preoperative planning of deep inferior epigastric artery perforator flap reconstruction with multislice-CT angiography: imaging findings and initial experience. J Plast Reconstr Aesthet Surg 2006;59:585–93.

13. Masia J, Clavero JA, Larrañaga JR, et al. Multidetector-row computed tomography in the planning of abdominal perforator flaps. J Plast Reconstr Aesthet Surg 2006;59:594–9.

14. Rozen WM, Ashton MW, Grinsell D, et al. Establishing the case for CT angiography in the preoperative imaging of abdominal wall perforators. Microsurgery 2008;28:306–13.

15. Rozen WM, Anavekar NS, Ashton MW, et al. Does the preoperative imaging of perforators with CT angiography improve operative outcomes in breast reconstruction? Microsurgery 2008;28:516–23.

16. Smit JM, Dimopoulou A, Liss AG, et al. Preoperative CT angiography reduces surgery time in perforator flap reconstruction. J Plast Reconstr Aesthet Surg 2009;62:1112–7.

17. Cina A, Salgarello M, Barone-Adesi L, et al. Planning breast reconstruction with deep inferior epigastric artery perforating vessels: multidetector CT angiography versus color Doppler US. Radiology 2010; 255:979–87.

18. Neil-Dwyer JG, Ludman CN, Schaverien M, et al. Magnetic resonance angiography in preoperative planning of deep inferior epigastric artery perforator flaps. J Plast Reconstr Aesthet Surg 2009;62:1661–5.

19. Cademartiri F, Mollet NR, van der Lugt A, et al. Intravenous contrast material administration at helical 16-detector row CT coronary angiography: effect of iodine concentration on vascular attenuation. Radiology 2005;236:661–5.

20. Becker CR, Hong C, Knez A, et al. Optimal contrast application for cardiac 4-detector-row computed tomography. Invest Radiol 2003;38:690–4.

21. Phillips TJ, Stella DL, Rozen WM, et al. Abdominal wall CT angiography: a detailed account of a newly established preoperative imaging technique. Radiology 2008;249:32–44.

22. Cademartiri F, Luccichenti G, van Der Lugt A, et al. Sixteen-row multislice computed tomography: basic concepts, protocols, and enhanced clinical applications. Semin Ultrasound CT MR 2004;25:2–16.

23. Alonso-Burgos A, García-Tutor E, Bastarrika G, et al. Preoperative planning of DIEP and SGAP flaps: preliminary experience with magnetic resonance angiography using 3-tesla equipment and blood-pool

contrast medium. J Plast Reconstr Aesthet Surg 2010; 63:298–304.

24. Greenspun D, Vasile J, Levine JL, et al. Anatomic imaging of abdominal perforator flaps without ionizing radiation: seeing is believing with magnetic resonance imaging angiography. J Reconstr Microsurg 2010;26:37–44.

25. Vasile JV, Newman T, Rusch DG, et al. Anatomic imaging of gluteal perforator flaps without ionizing radiation: seeing is believing with magnetic resonance angiography. J Reconstr Microsurg 2010;26:45–57.

26. Masia J, Kosutic D, Cervelli D, et al. In search of the ideal method in perforator mapping: noncontrast magnetic resonance imaging. J Reconstr Microsurg 2010;26:29–35.

27. Schaverien M, Saint-Cyr M, Arbique G, et al. Arterial and venous anatomies of the deep inferior epigastric perforator and superficial inferior epigastric artery flaps. Plast Reconstr Surg 2008;121:1909–19.

28. Clavero JA, Masia J, Larrañaga J, et al. MDCT in the preoperative planning of abdominal perforator surgery for postmastectomy breast reconstruction. AJR Am J Roentgenol 2008;191:670–6.

29. Masia J, Larrañaga J, Clavero JA, et al. The value of the multidetector row computed tomography for the preoperative planning of deep inferior epigastric artery perforator flap: our experience in 162 cases. Ann Plast Surg 2008;60:29–36.

30. Rozen WM, Murray AC, Ashton MW, et al. The cutaneous course of deep inferior epigastric perforators: implications for flap thinning. J Plast Reconstr Aesthet Surg 2009;62:986–90.

31. Pacifico MD, See MS, Cavale N, et al. Preoperative planning for DIEP breast reconstruction: early experience of the use of computerised tomography angiography with VoNavix 3D software for perforator navigation. J Plast Reconstr Aesthet Surg 2009;62: 1464–9.

32. Whitaker IS, Rozen WM, Smit JM, et al. Peritoneocutaneous perforators in deep inferior epigastric perforator flaps: a cadaveric dissection and computed tomographic angiography study. Microsurgery 2009;29:124–7.

33. Rozen WM, Stella DL, Bowden J, et al. Advances in the pre-operative planning of deep inferior epigastric artery perforator flaps: magnetic resonance angiography. Microsurgery 2009;29:119–23.

34. Kim EK, Kang BS, Hong JP. The distribution of the perforators in the anterolateral thigh and the utility of multidetector row computed tomography angiography in preoperative planning. Ann Plast Surg 2010;65:155–60.

35. Chen SY, Lin WC, Deng SC, et al. Assessment of the perforators of anterolateral thigh flaps using 64-section multidetector computed tomographic angiography in head and neck cancer reconstruction. Eur J Surg Oncol 2010.

36. Ghattaura A, Henton J, Jallali N, et al. One hundred cases of abdominal-based free flaps in breast reconstruction. The impact of preoperative computed tomographic angiography. J Plast Reconstr Aesthet Surg 2010;63:1597–601.

37. Zhang Q, Qiao Q, Yang X, et al. Clinical application of the anterolateral thigh flap for soft tissue reconstruction. J Reconstr Microsurg 2010;26:87–94.

38. Visscher K, Boyd K, Ross DC, et al. Refining perforator selection for DIEP breast reconstruction using transit time flow volume measurements. J Reconstr Microsurg 2010;26:285–90.

39. Katz RD, Manahan MA, Rad AN, et al. Classification schema for anatomic variations of the inferior epigastric vasculature evaluated by abdominal CT angiograms for breast reconstruction. Microsurgery 2010;30(8):593–602.

40. Ting JW, Rozen WM, Leong J, et al. Free deep circumflex iliac artery vascularised bone flap for reconstruction of the distal radius: planning with CT angiography. Microsurgery 2010;30:163–7.

41. Rad AN, Flores JI, Prucz RB, et al. Clinical experience with the lateral septocutaneous superior gluteal artery perforator flap for autologous breast reconstruction. Microsurgery 2010;30:339–47.

42. Gacto-Sánchez P, Sicilia-Castro D, Gómez-Cía T, et al. Use of a three-dimensional virtual reality model for preoperative imaging in DIEP flap breast reconstruction. J Surg Res 2010;162:140–7.

43. Ribuffo D, Atzeni M, Saba L, et al. Clinical study of peroneal artery perforators with computed tomographic angiography: implications for fibular flap harvest. Surg Radiol Anat 2010;32:329–34.

Computed Tomographic Angiography: Clinical Applications

Warren M. Rozen, MBBS, BMedSc, PGDipSurgAnat, PhD*,
Daniel Chubb, MBBS(Hons), BMedSc,
Damien Grinsell, MBBS, FRACS,
Mark W. Ashton, MBBS, MD, FRACS

KEYWORDS

- CTA • Imaging • Perforator flap • Free flap
- Breast reconstruction

The use of preoperative imaging for planning free flap operations has been enthusiastically received by most reconstructive surgeons, with advances in both operative techniques and imaging techniques highlighting the benefits of such imaging. Computed tomographic angiography (CTA) in particular, has emerged as a beneficial aid in the planning of perforator flaps, with proven efficacy in improving operative outcomes and allowing for accurate and appropriate preoperative decision making.[1–4] Its role has emerged for many perforator flap operations, and many centers have now published large series of data to show these outcomes. In addition to modifying flap planning, preoperative imaging has been explored as a means to planning the optimal mode of dissection and to minimize donor site morbidity. With further technological improvements in imaging techniques, these aims have become increasingly realized.

In its role for preoperative planning, CTA is able to detect perforators at any potential donor site, and with modern high-resolution scanners allows for detection of almost all vessels more than 0.3 mm in size.[2,3] This accuracy makes CTA the most accurate technology currently available for the preoperative mapping of perforators. In addition to this accuracy, CTA is able to evaluate more than 1 potential donor site simultaneously, allowing the surgeon flexibility in donor site selection as well as perforator selection within a single scan.

Perforator flap surgery is currently a mainstay in the management of breast reconstruction, with a range of donor sites commonly used for both partial and total breast reconstruction. Given the potential for overall improvements in both flap vascularity and survival, as well as donor site morbidity, a range of applications of CTA in the setting of autologous breast reconstruction have emerged. These applications include donor site selection, flap selection, and perforator selection for free tissue transfer, as well as flap and perforator selection for locoregional perforator flap options. Other applications for CTA that have become useful include the appraisal of recipient vessels for free tissue transfer and the screening for comorbidities, such as metastatic disease or

Disclosure Statement: The authors all confirm that there are no any actual or potential conflicts of interest, including employment, consultancies, stock ownership, honoraria, patent applications/registrations, and grants or other funding.
Conflicts of Interest: None.
The Taylor Laboratory, Jack Brockhoff Reconstructive Plastic Surgery Research Unit, Department of Anatomy and Cell Biology, The University of Melbourne, Room E533, Grattan Street, Parkville, Victoria 3050, Australia
* Corresponding author.
E-mail address: warrenrozen@hotmail.com

Clin Plastic Surg 38 (2011) 229–239
doi:10.1016/j.cps.2011.03.007

incidental findings that may influence operative care. These and other useful techniques are explored in this article.

TECHNIQUE

The process of scanning a patient to obtain images that can be used for preoperative planning is not complicated,[5] and a range of scanning protocols can be used to achieve equally good visualization of perforators. In general, the aim is to achieve arterial phase scans, which eliminate venous contamination, avoid confusion between different structures, and maximize arterial filling. We thus recommend triggering the scan from the origin of the pedicle, and scanning in the direction of blood flow through the perforating vessels. For example, for deep inferior epigastric artery perforator (DIEP) flaps, the scan is triggered from the external iliac/common femoral artery junction and the scan is performed in a caudocranial direction. This technique is modified for each donor site.

Analysis of CTA images can similarly be performed using a range of techniques, with the raw scan data through axial slices able to show all of the important information; however, visual appreciation of the vascular anatomy is best achieved with the use of software-generated three-dimensional (3D) reconstructions. These reconstructions are easy to interpret by surgeons and show the anatomic relationships of each vessel in a single 3D image. There are a variety of software applications that are able to generate suitable images for operative planning. Each generated image can be saved for reference during the operation, with only several images required for easy intraoperative reference. Rather than referral to a radiologist for all image analysis, we have found that many surgeons prefer to see or generate the 3D reconstructions themselves, because appreciation of the 3D course of a perforator on a saved image can be difficult.

FREE FLAP DONOR SITES

Preoperative imaging of a donor site with CTA can achieve 2 global aims: first, to confirm that a proposed donor site is suitable in that role, and second, to select the most appropriate vasculature from that donor site as the basis of flap design. All potential donor sites for free flap breast reconstruction can be investigated with CTA to determine the exact nature of their vasculature. A variety of potential donor sites have been used for autologous breast reconstruction, with many of these still in widespread use; however, the anterior abdominal wall has remained the first choice

because of the superior cosmesis of its donor site. Abdominal wall flaps used in this role include the free transverse rectus abdominis myocutaneous (TRAM) flap, muscle-sparing variants of the TRAM flap, the DIEP flap, and the superficial inferior epigastric artery (SIEA) flap. Although the abdominal wall is versatile and suitable in most cases, several other free flap donor sites are suitable as first-line or particularly where the abdominal wall is unsuitable (eg, if there is scarring). These sites include the superior and inferior gluteal artery perforator flaps (SGAPs and IGAPs, respectively) and the transverse upper gracilis (TUG) flap.

Anterior Abdominal Wall Flaps (TRAM, DIEP, and SIEA Flaps)

Free flaps based on the lower anterior abdominal wall integument have progressed in techniques in a donor-site–sparing fashion, which has simultaneously increased surgical complexity and decision making. From inclusion of all deep inferior epigastric artery (DIEA) perforators in the TRAM flap, to the selection of the optimal perforators in the DIEP flap, preoperative imaging can substantially improve decision-making ability. For the SIEA flap, where anatomic variation is widespread and a suitable SIEA is present in only 10% of patients, preoperative planning is of utmost importance.[6,7] The abdominal wall vasculature is highly variable, potentially more than most other body regions. The DIEAs originate from the external iliac artery, and ascend within the rectus sheath on the deep surface of rectus abdominis, distributing musculocutaneous perforators to supply the overlying integument. Perforator variability is not only in location but also in size and course. The ability of this anatomy to cause operative havoc led to the use of the external Doppler prove for perforator mapping from the early days of such surgery. However, with low sensitivity and specificity in this role, the development of advanced perforator imaging technique arose in response to this uncertainty.

For perforator mapping in the anterior abdominal wall, CTA has become established as the gold standard, shown to be highly accurate in both cadaveric and clinical studies, with a sensitivity and specificity in such mapping approaching 100%.[2,8] It has been shown to accurately identify the DIEA (**Fig. 1**), all of its major branches, and its musculocutaneous perforating branches. In addition to the location and size of these vessels, a 3D appreciation of the course of the perforators can be shown (**Fig. 2**). The relative dominance of the superficial arterial system can also be determined (**Fig. 3**). The use of CTA to show this

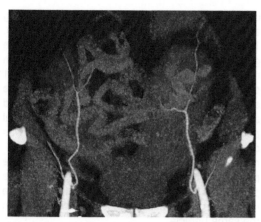

Fig. 1. Computed tomographic angiogram (CTA) of the anterior abdominal wall vasculature, demonstrating the opacified deep inferior epigastric arteries.

anatomy can directly aid selection of the hemiabdominal wall of choice for dissection, the approximate volume of tissue supplied per perforator, and the perforators of choice for supply to the flap. CTA has been compared with other modalities such as color duplex (ecocolor Doppler) ultrasonography and magnetic resonance angiography (MRA),[9] with superior results in such studies. Furthermore, improvements in outcomes have been shown with statistical significance, with faster dissection times and reduced operating times, improved flap vascularity and survival, and improved donor site morbidity all shown.[4] These

benefits have propelled CTA into increasingly widespread use. A wealth of information is gained from an abdominal wall CTA that contributes to the superior advantage of this modality. Not only does an abdominal wall CTA show the DIEA and its branches, but it also shows other vessels supplying the abdominal wall, including the SIEA, superficial superior epigastric artery, deep superior epigastric artery, deep circumflex iliac artery, superficial circumflex iliac artery, intercostal arteries (lateral and posterior), and lumbar arteries. The SGA and IGA are also shown within the same scan range, offering consideration of alternative donor site options. In addition to the vasculature (which can rarely show abdominal wall perforators coming from a direct intra-abdominal source vessel), the soft tissues and fascial layers of the abdominal wall and the abdominal contents are also included within the scan data. The use of all of this information can directly assist and change operative planning.

There are significant differences in scanning protocols between abdominal wall perforator CTA and routine abdominal CTA. Without these changes, perforators are not adequately imaged and scans are unlikely to be suitable or worthwhile. Our usual protocol requires adequate positioning of the patient (to match the supine operative position) without compressive clothing, and scanning the range of the flap only (pubic symphysis to 4 cm above the umbilicus). We scan at the level of the common femoral artery and trigger the scan

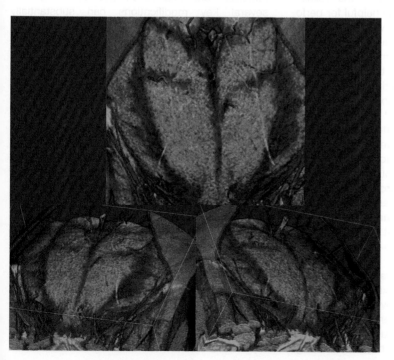

Fig. 2. Computed tomographic angiogram (CTA) of the anterior abdominal wall vasculature, demonstrating the subcutaneous course of each deep inferior epigastric artery (DIEA) perforator can easily be assessed. This is a volume rendered technique (VRT) reconstruction, with axial maximum intensity projection (MIP) images used to determine sub- and intramuscular courses.

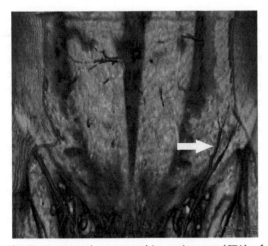

Fig. 3. Computed tomographic angiogram (CTA) of the anterior abdominal wall vasculature. While there is a large (dominant) periumbilical perforator on the right, there is a relative paucity of deep inferior epigastric artery (DIEA) perforators on the left side associated with a large superficial inferior epigastric artery (SIEA) (*arrow*).

when it opacifies to greater than 100 Hounsfield units (HU), scanning the patient in the caudocranial direction (to match filling of the DIEA).

GAP Flaps

The gluteal region provides a highly advantageous donor site for autologous breast reconstruction, with good available flap volume and reliable vasculature.[10–13] Just as CTA is helpful for perforator imaging in the abdominal wall, so too can it show the vasculature of the gluteal region. CTA can allow for choice of the optimal flap and donor vessel (SGA vs IGA); choice of the optimal perforator within that flap; optimization of flap design and orientation to create a more aesthetic scar position. Often SGAP and IGAP flaps are planned with the use of multiple perforators, and CTA can select those perforators that can minimize muscle sacrifice between selected perforators.

CTA can show the entire course of the donor vasculature, from regional source to skin (**Figs. 4** and **5**). The SGA is the largest branch of the internal iliac artery, originating as the continuation of the posterior division of that vessel. It passes out of the pelvis through the greater sciatic foramen and divides almost immediately into deep and superficial branches. The superficial branch enters the gluteus maximus on its deep surface, and often divides several times within this muscle, sending multiple perforators to supply the skin over the gluteus maximus and the sacrum. The angiosome extends well beyond the edge

of the gluteus maximus, and most prefer taking a more lateral flap to gain extra perforator length. The branching pattern of the SGA within the gluteus maximus is extremely variable, and can make it difficult to raise the flap on more than 1 perforator if the anatomy is not known before surgery. Previously, some investigators advocated a single perforator for the flap, with additional perforators selected if favorable anatomy was discovered intraoperatively. It has been our experience that CTA almost always allows for multiple perforators to be selected if wanted, and for those perforators to be traced on imaging to their source (virtual surgery), ensuring that they originate from the same pedicle.

The IGA arises as one of the terminal branches of the anterior division of the internal iliac artery. It also passes through the greater sciatic foramen to exit the pelvis, although unlike the SGA, it runs inferior to the piriformis. Although its main course is to descend in the interval between the greater trochanter and the ischial tuberosity, it sends a few perforating branches to supply the inferior portion of the gluteus maximus and the overlying skin, a zone of supply just inferior to the primary angiosome of the SGA. The intramuscular dissection of these perforators is difficult, and preoperative awareness gained by CTA can be indispensable in selecting those with shorter intramuscular and partially septocutaneous courses.

The standard scan used to assess DIEA perforators can be used to visualize the SGAP and IGAP; however, our experience has identified that several key modifications can substantially improve the scan quality. First, triggering the scan at the source pedicle (the internal iliac artery) maximizes arterial filling of the gluteal artery perforators. In addition, these scans are performed in the prone position, to avoid pressure distortion of the gluteal soft-tissue and vascular anatomy.

TUG Flaps

The TUG flap has emerged as another useful donor site, and in some centers this flap has become the standard.[14,15] The TUG flap is a free flap usually consisting of a segment of the proximal gracilis muscle and up to a 25-cm × 10-cm skin paddle oriented transversely (although a vertical paddle has been used too).[16] The vascular pedicle of the TUG flap is the descending branch of the medial circumflex femoral artery, generally with 2 venae comitantes, yielding a pedicle about 6 cm long. This flap may also be raised as a perforator flap if the anatomy is favorable. This flap is favored by some because of its reported low donor site morbidity.

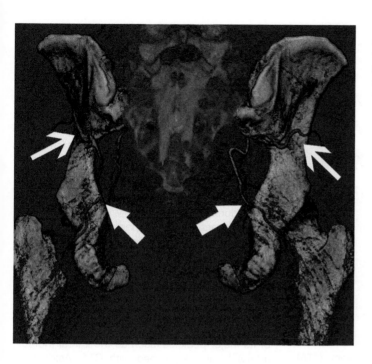

Fig. 4. Computed tomographic angiogram (CTA) of the gluteal vasculature, with thin arrows highlighting the superior gluteal vessels while thick arrows show the inferior gluteal vessels.

Imaging with CTA can clearly show the source vasculature and perforator anatomy (**Fig. 6**). This characteristic can enable accurate flap planning and design of the skin paddle and aid in consideration of muscle-sparing procedures. The scanning technique for this flap (or any limb perforator flap)

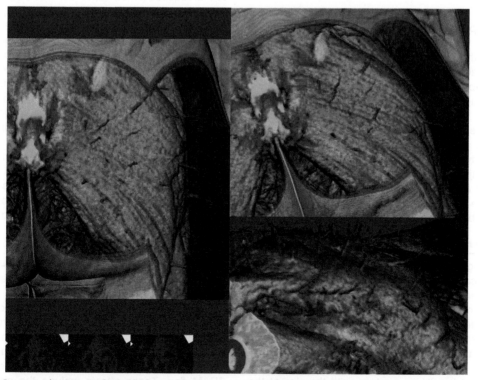

Fig. 5. Computed tomographic angiogram (CTA), volume rendered technique (VRT) reconstruction for the same patient as **Fig. 4**. Several large superior gluteal artery (SGA) perforators can be seen. These images also demonstrate the zone of flap and skin supplied by the perforator, allowing for optimal flap design.

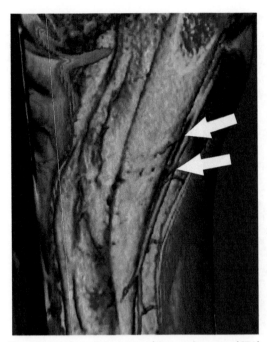

Fig. 6. Computed tomographic angiogram (CTA), volume rendered technique (VRT) reconstruction of the lower limb, demonstrating gracilis perforators (*arrows*) mapped in the planning of a transverse upper gracilis (TUG) flap. This is a medial view of the left thigh, with anterior to the right of the image.

is simple: we place the patient in the position in which the flap will be raised, trigger the scan from the origin of the source vessel (common femoral artery), and scan in a proximal-distal direction. The gracilis muscle can clearly be shown on imaging, and perforators (either septocutaneous or musculocutaneous) through or around the muscle can be highlighted. The intraflap course of the perforators delineated on CTA has also confirmed the clinical and surgical findings that the major orientation/direction of the gracilis perforators (ie, their angiosome) is a transverse skin paddle as opposed to the vertical skin paddle described earlier.

Lumbar Artery Perforator Flaps

Although not a common candidate as a donor site for reconstruction, the lumbar region does offer a potential donor site for breast reconstruction, and lumbar artery perforators have been used in this role. Lumbar perforating arteries segmentally supply the lumbar skin, usually as fasciocutaneous perforators between the erector spinae and quadratus lumborum muscles.[17,18] Each lumbar segment has its own artery, with the size of the vessels increasing inferiorly. To obtain a reasonable pedicle length for breast reconstruction

deep dissection between erector spinae and quadratus lumborum is required.

The size and distribution of lumbar artery perforators have been studied with cadaveric angiographic techniques, and CTA has been used previously to determine the vascular anatomy of a particular patient to help improve the selection of pedicles and flap design.[17]

LOCOREGIONAL FLAP DONOR SITES

Autologous breast reconstruction can be achieved with a range of locoregional options, with the latissimus dorsi and pedicle-TRAM flap comprising the main players. Similarly, partial or small-volume total breast reconstruction can be achieved with a variety of other locoregional flaps.[19] These include the thoracodorsal artery perforator (TAP/TDAP) flap and internal mammary artery perforator (IMAP) flaps. Breast-sharing techniques using pedicled mammary tissue on internal mammary perforators[20] or even as free flaps based on one of its major pedicles (such as the lateral thoracic artery)[21] can be planned with CTA. Aside from the TRAM flap, each of these other locoregional options is based on the vasculature of the thoracic wall, and can be visualized using routine chest CTA, because the timing of such scans is identical to that required (timed from the thoracic aorta). It is often necessary to incorporate a small (approximately 5-second) delay between opacification of the aortic arch and commencement of the scan to allow the contrast to completely fill the perforators. Because all of these flaps can be imaged with a single scan, it is possible to use CTA to select the locoregional pedicle of choice as well as to select the best perforator for flap design. The major limitation of thoracic CTA is the relative proximity of the scan range to remaining breast tissue (which is at a higher than normal risk for recurrent or new malignancy) and to the thyroid gland, when compared with more distal scanning. As such, benefits from the use of such imaging should be weighed up against the risks, and selected on an individualized basis.

Pedicled TRAM Flaps

The pedicled TRAM flap has been a mainstay for autologous breast reconstruction for 30 years, and is still among the most commonly used pedicled flap options for breast reconstruction. Although imaging of the anterior abdominal wall has already been discussed, CTA can achieve several key effects in the planning of a pedicled TRAM flap. These effects include the ability of CTA to show the relative vascularity of each abdominal wall zone, and thus define the safe zones for inclusion within the flap, as well as defining the zone of rectus muscle containing the dominant DIEA perforators, and thus enabling consideration of a muscle-splitting or muscle-sparing option.

An additional tool for CTA has been to monitor for the effects of the delay phenomenon (surgically or otherwise) in TRAM flaps.[22] Surgical delay of the pedicled TRAM flap has been widely used to improve flap vascularity, and particularly its venous drainage, and with the use of CTA, dilatation of choke zones can be made apparent, confirming the success of such techniques, and enabling safe surgery. CTA images showing this phenomenon have been previously published.[22]

IMAP Flaps

The internal mammary artery distributes multiple perforating branches that traverse the anterior thoracic wall. Almost all of these branches closely overlie its position approximately 1 finger's breadth from the lateral edge of the sternum. The perforators pass through the intercostal spaces, in the upper part of the space, and supply the area of skin above the sternum as well as the superomedial parenchyma and skin of the breast. These perforators can often be used for either small local flaps or as recipient vessels for a free flap. Although IMAP flaps can generally only be small volume, they may be useful in partial or low-volume reconstructions.[23] A major difficulty with IMAP flaps is the unpredictability of perforator size and location. Although larger perforators generally traverse the upper spaces, this is highly variable. CTA can readily delineate the exact position and caliber of each of these perforators, allowing for the preoperative assessment of feasibility of this flap, as well as optimizing perforator selection and flap design (**Fig. 7**).

Intercostal Artery Perforator Flaps

Intercostal vessels enter their respective intercostal spaces both anteriorly and posteriorly. The posterior intercostal arteries are supplied by the costocervical trunk (upper 2 spaces) or the thoracic aorta (remaining 9 spaces), whereas the anterior intercostal spaces are supplied by the internal mammary/thoracic artery (upper 6 spaces) or the musculophrenic artery (in the 3 spaces below). The anterior and posterior intercostal arteries anastomose in an end-to-end fashion. Each of the anterior and posterior intercostal arteries distributes perforators to supply the overlying skin, forming the basis for posterior intercostal artery perforator flaps and anterior intercostal artery perforator flaps. These vessels also give rise to a lateral cutaneous branch, which perforates the thoracic wall and forms a large part of the cutaneous blood supply of the lateral thoracic wall (lateral intercostal artery perforator flaps). Although these classically arise just anterior to the border of latissimus dorsi, they are variable

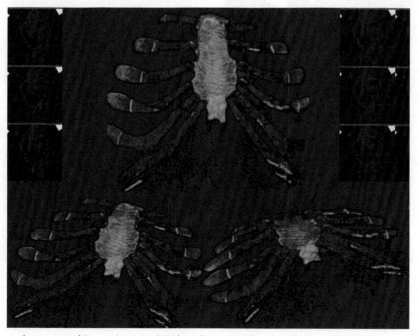

Fig. 7. Computed tomographic angiogram (CTA), volume rendered technique (VRT) images of the internal mammary artery and its perforators. Bilateral second space perforators can be seen.

in their size and location. The skin territory of this pedicle lies between the posterior axillary line and the midline of the abdomen, and may include an area of 3 to 5 intercostal segments.

Intercostal artery perforator flaps are typically small volume, but may be used for partial reconstructions, particularly where the tissue defect is in the lateral part of the breast.[24] CTA allows the surgeon to determine the exact position and caliber of all of the intercostal perforators before dissection begins, allowing flap selection, perforator selection, and flap design decisions to be made in a way that optimizes flap vasculature (**Fig. 8**).

TAP/TDAP Flaps

Although the latissimus dorsi flap can be used for breast reconstruction, harvest of this muscle may lead to substantial donor site morbidity. The TAP flap allows the surgeon to use the same vasculature to perform a free or pedicled flap for breast reconstruction,[20] although the TAP flap is typically of a lower volume and slightly shorter pedicle length than the classic latissimus dorsi flap. The

usefulness of the TAP flap is usually limited to low-volume and partial breast reconstructions. The thoracodorsal artery arises from the subscapular artery shortly after that vessel arises from the axillary artery. It travels inferiorly alongside the thoracodorsal nerve to enter the latissimus dorsi on its deep surface, supplying the overlying skin via musculocutaneous perforators. Shortly before it courses beneath the muscle, it frequently gives off 1 or more fasciocutaneous perforators that can be found on the anterior border of latissimus dorsi. These perforators in particular form the basis of the TAP flap, and CTA is reliable at detecting the presence, size, and location of these perforators, allowing the surgeon confidence in the operation, as well as in their flap design (**Fig. 9**).

RECIPIENT SITES

Although the more commonly accepted role for preoperative imaging in autologous breast reconstruction is for donor site assessment, it is also possible to use CTA to assess the recipient site. Given the limited number of potential recipient sites on the chest wall, and the anatomic variation of the region, such imaging can have a substantial effect on predicting operative success. Recipient vessel

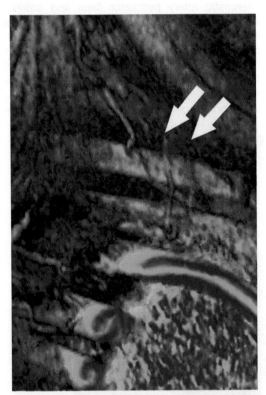

Fig. 8. Computed tomographic angiogram (CTA), volume rendered technique (VRT) image of the chest wall, highlighting lateral cutaneous branches of the intercostal arteries (*arrows*). This image is of the right lateral thoracic wall, with latissimus dorsi (partially cropped) on the left of the image, and the right of the image being anterior.

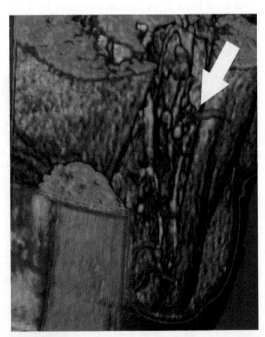

Fig. 9. Computed tomographic angiogram (CTA), volume rendered technique (VRT) image of the chest wall, highlighting a thoracodorsal artery perforator (*thick arrow*). This image is of the left thoracic wall, viewed from anteriorly. The fasciocutaneous perforator is wrapping around the anterior border of latissimus dorsi to supply the overlying skin.

flow is the primary source of blood supply to a free flap, and so it is important that this vessel is of sufficient caliber and has appropriate regional anatomy. This characteristic is particularly important where the recipient vessel may have been affected by trauma or radiotherapy, as in the case of previous breast surgery and/or radiotherapy. A single CTA of the chest wall is able to assess all of the potential recipient sites in the area, and determine their location and caliber (**Fig. 10**).

The internal mammary, thoracodorsal, and circumflex scapula arteries are the most commonly used recipient vessels. Their anatomy is well known, and they are usually of sufficient size for microvascular anastomosis. Imaging of the internal mammary artery can be made difficult by the density of surrounding tissues, and adjustments of the 3D reconstructions through their color look-up tables or cropping of surrounding tissues from the 3D image may be necessary to produce an image that allows useful interpretation. Scan timing can also be modified to enable accurate visualization of the venous anatomy. The thoracodorsal vessels are sometimes obscured if a CTA is taken with the patient in the anatomic position, and the position of the artery varies with movement of the upper limb. Careful consideration of these issues is warranted before performing a CTA of the chest, particularly for evaluation of the thoracodorsal artery.

In considering the option for imaging recipient sites with CTA, the risks of radiation dosage must be weighed up against the benefits of the scan. Radiation dosage is of a substantially greater concern in the region of the chest wall when compared with the lower abdominal wall. Although CTA of the chest wall does not necessarily expose the patient to a greater overall radiation dose than a CTA of the abdominal wall,[25] the radiation to this region is more of a problem for several reasons. First, the radiation is nearer to radiosensitive structures such as the thymus and thyroid glands. Second, there is a greater exposure of any residual breast tissue to this radiation, and this is in the context that most patients requiring autologous breast reconstruction have already had at least 1 breast cancer. A further reason is that this radiation exposure is in addition to radiation already received during the initial perforator imaging scan.

In our experience, CTA imaging of the recipient vessels has a low likelihood of changing the operative plan in most patients, and there is no clearly shown clinical benefit to imaging these vessels. These vessels are usually easily mapped with non-irradiating techniques such as duplex/Doppler sonography. Given the higher risks and lower benefits of this scan, the balance may be tilted toward not performing such an investigation in most patients. However, any decision to perform this test must be made on an individual basis, and there certainly may be situations in which this application becomes useful.

OTHER APPLICATIONS

The use of a CT scan for a specific purpose does not rule out the finding of incidentalomas, or incidental findings not specifically sought. In abdominal scans, many such findings have been reported, including adrenal masses, liver lesions, and renal artery stenoses. More importantly, cases have been reported in which previously unidentified metastatic disease has been discovered. In the setting of a preoperative scan, many such findings can have profound implications for surgery, and we believe this is an added benefit of such preoperative imaging. For this reason, some units that perform scans for the purpose of operative planning also have the images reported by a radiologist to specifically look for such incidental findings. Follow-up of these findings may not be mandatory, and varies depending on the nature of the problem identified.

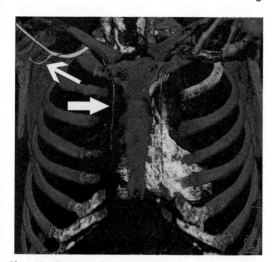

Fig. 10. Computed tomographic angiogram (CTA), volume rendered technique (VRT) reconstruction of the chest wall, showing potential recipient vessels for a free flap. The internal mammary artery (*thick arrow*) is visualised by cropping away the costal cartilage. The subscapular artery (*thin arrow*) can be seen branching into its thoracodorsal and circumflex scapular components.

SUMMARY

CTA can offer the reconstructive surgeon a range of clinical applications, regardless of the reconstructive problem or selected technique in autologous breast reconstruction. From local to free flaps, donor site to recipient site, CTA can aid operative planning and improve outcomes.

A concluding note on the implementation of this technology into clinical practice is vital, with an inadequately reported scan paramount to a needless or wasted procedure. We have found that the most effective way to produce images that are intuitive for the surgeon is to produce multicolor 3D reconstructions of the area of interest, which can then be rotated and modified to display the relevant anatomy. Many programs are able to produce satisfactory 3D reconstructions from the raw data (standard DICOM [Digital Imaging and Communications in Medicine] files). We have used both Osirix (Osirix Medical Imaging Software, GPL Licensing Open Source Initiative) and Syngo InSpace (Siemens Syngo InSpace 4D, version 2006A; Siemens Medical Solutions, Erlangen, Germany), and have been able to produce excellent images with both programs (Osirix is available for free online). In addition, we have experimented with image-guided stereotaxy with great success, but do not use this as part of our routine practice. Because these scans are performed to assist with surgical decision making, the 3D images are initially analyzed by a member of the surgical team, ensuring a smooth transition from scanner to patient.

REFERENCES

1. Rozen WM, Ashton MW, Whitaker IS, et al. The financial implications of computed tomographic angiography in DIEP flap surgery: a cost analysis. Microsurgery 2009;29:168–9.
2. Rozen WM, Ashton MW, Stella DL, et al. The accuracy of computed tomographic angiography for mapping the perforators of the deep inferior epigastric artery: a blinded, prospective cohort study. Plast Reconstr Surg 2008;122:1003–9.
3. Rozen WM, Ashton MW, Grinsell D, et al. Establishing the case for CT angiography in the preoperative imaging of abdominal wall perforators. Microsurgery 2008;28:306–13.
4. Rozen WM, Anavekar NS, Ashton MW, et al. Does the preoperative imaging of perforators with CT angiography improve operative outcomes in breast reconstruction? Microsurgery 2008;28:516–23.
5. Rozen WM, Phillips TJ, Stella DL, et al. Preoperative CT angiography for DIEP flaps: 'must-have' lessons for the radiologist. J Plast Reconstr Aesthet Surg 2009;62:e650–1.
6. Rozen WM, Chubb D, Grinsell D, et al. The variability of the Superficial Inferior Epigastric Artery (SIEA) and its angiosome: a clinical anatomical study. Microsurgery 2010;30:386–91.
7. Rozen WM, Chubb D, Grinsell D, et al. The SIEA angiosome: interindividual variability predicted preoperatively. Plast Reconstr Surg 2009;124:327–8 [author reply: 328–30].
8. Rozen WM, Ashton MW, Stella DL, et al. The accuracy of computed tomographic angiography for mapping the perforators of the DIEA: a cadaveric study. Plast Reconstr Surg 2008;122:363–9.
9. Rozen WM, Stella DL, Bowden J, et al. Advances in the pre-operative planning of deep inferior epigastric artery perforator flaps: magnetic resonance angiography. Microsurgery 2009;29:119–23.
10. Baumeister S, Werdin F, Peek A. The sGAP flap: rare exception or second choice in autologous breast reconstruction? J Reconstr Microsurg 2010;26:251–8.
11. Rozen WM, Ting JW, Grinsell D, et al. Superior and inferior gluteal artery perforators: in-vivo anatomical study and planning for breast reconstruction. J Plast Reconstr Aesthet Surg 2011;64(2):217–25.
12. Guerra AB, Metzinger SE, Bidros RS, et al. Breast reconstruction with gluteal artery perforator (GAP) flaps: a critical analysis of 142 cases. Ann Plast Surg 2004;52:118–25.
13. Guerra AB, Soueid N, Metzinger SE, et al. Simultaneous bilateral breast reconstruction with superior gluteal artery perforator (SGAP) flaps. Ann Plast Surg 2004;53:305–10.
14. Arnez ZM, Pogorelec D, Planinsek F, et al. Breast reconstruction by the free transverse gracilis (TUG) flap. Br J Plast Surg 2004;57:20–6.
15. Fansa H, Schirmer S, Warnecke IC, et al. The transverse myocutaneous gracilis muscle flap: a fast and reliable method for breast reconstruction. Plast Reconstr Surg 2008;122:1326–33.
16. Kind GM, Foster RD. The longitudinal gracilis myocutaneous flap: broadening options in breast reconstruction. Ann Plast Surg 2008;61:513–20.
17. Kiil BJ, Rozen WM, Pan WR, et al. The lumbar artery perforators: a cadaveric and clinical anatomical study. Plast Reconstr Surg 2009;123:1229–38.
18. de Weerd L, Elvenes OP, Strandenes E, et al. Autologous breast reconstruction with a free lumbar artery perforator flap. Br J Plast Surg 2003;56:180–3.
19. Losken A, Hamdi M. Partial breast reconstruction: current perspectives. Plast Reconstr Surg 2009;124:722–36.
20. Hamdi M, Salgarello M, Barone-Adesi L, et al. Use of the thoracodorsal artery perforator (TDAP) flap with implant in breast reconstruction. Ann Plast Surg 2008;61:143–6.
21. Morritt AN, Grinsell D, Morrison WA. Postmastectomy breast reconstruction using a microvascular breast-sharing technique. Plast Reconstr Surg 2006;118:1313–6 [discussion: 1317–9].
22. Ribuffo D, Atzeni M, Corrias F, et al. Preoperative Angio-CT preliminary study of the TRAM flap after selective vascular delay. Ann Plast Surg 2007;59:611–6.

23. Saint-Cyr M, Schaverien M, Rohrich RJ. Preexpanded second intercostal space internal mammary artery pedicle perforator flap: case report and anatomical study. Plast Reconstr Surg 2009;123:1659–64.

24. Hamdi M, Van Landuyt K, Blondeel P, et al. Autologous breast augmentation with the lateral intercostal artery perforator flap in massive weight loss patients. J Plast Reconstr Aesthet Surg 2009;62: 65–70.

25. Rozen WM, Whitaker IS, Stella DL, et al. The radiation exposure of Computed Tomographic Angiography (CTA) in DIEP flap planning: low dose but high impact. J Plast Reconstr Aesthet Surg 2009; 62:e654–5.

Computed Tomographic Angiography: Assessing Outcomes

William J. Casey III, MD*, Alanna M. Rebecca, MD,
Peter A. Kreymerman, MD, Luis H. Macias, MD

KEYWORDS

- CT angiography • Deep inferior epigastric perforator flap
- DIEP

The benefits of autologous breast reconstruction are well established, particularly in individuals who have failed implant-based reconstruction or require adjuvant radiation.[1] Multiple donor sites are available, providing an abundance of soft tissue similar in texture to the original breast. A natural breast contour can be achieved while avoiding future problems associated with prosthetic, implant-based techniques, such as capsular contracture, implant malposition, or implant rupture. The description of the pedicled transverse rectus abdominis musculocutaneous (TRAM) flap by Hartrampf and colleagues[2] revolutionized breast reconstruction, allowing for total autologous reconstruction with vascularized soft tissue in a single stage. The lower abdomen has since become the preferred donor site for breast reconstruction for surgeons performing autologous procedures.[1,3–8] A growing body of literature detailing the anatomy of the integument of the anterior abdominal wall and its underlying source vessels has led to refinements in operative techniques designed to maximize the reconstructive result while minimizing donor site morbidity.[9–20]

PERFORATOR FLAPS

In 1967, Fujino[21] reported that the contribution of perforators to the interstitial fluid turnover in axial flaps is approximately equal to the contribution made by the axial artery itself. Twenty years later, Taylor and Palmer[22] performed an anatomic study of human angiosomes and found an average of 374 musculocutaneous and septocutaneous perforators larger than 0.5 mm throughout the body. The perforator flap concept was introduced by Kroll and Rosenfield[23] in 1988, and 1 year later Koshima and Soeda[24] reported 2 abdominal perforator-based flaps to reconstruct a groin and tongue defect, coining the term perforator flap. The deep inferior epigastric artery perforator (DIEP) flap has since gained widespread acceptance as one of the ideal methods of breast reconstruction after its introduction by Allen[25] in 1994. The superficial inferior epigastric artery (SIEA) flap represents the least invasive means of transferring the lower abdominal skin and fat, requiring no dissection within the muscle or fascia. However, the SIEA may not be available in many cases, is not as reliable across the midline, and may have a higher incidence of arterial thrombosis.[26]

The major disadvantage of these flaps is that they can be difficult to harvest. Furthermore, although refinements in the technique have led to improvements in donor site morbidity, there seems to be an inverse relationship between donor site morbidity and flap-specific complications related to flap perfusion.[27] In other words, although donor site morbidity is reduced to a minimum, flap reliability and perfusion can be adversely affected to

The authors have nothing to disclose.
Division of Plastic and Reconstructive Surgery, Mayo Clinic in Arizona, 5777 East Mayo Boulevard, Phoenix, AZ 85054, USA
* Corresponding author.
E-mail address: Casey.williamjoseph@mayo.edu

Clin Plastic Surg 38 (2011) 241–252
doi:10.1016/j.cps.2011.03.003

some degree. In a study of 179 patients, Wu and colleagues[28] demonstrated that the patients perceived a reduced duration of postoperative pain and had improved postoperative abdominal strength when undergoing less-invasive procedures (muscle-sparing TRAM [MS-TRAM] vs DIEP vs SIEA). In this study, DIEP flaps were statistically similar to SIEA flaps. In a meta-analysis of free TRAM and DIEP flaps, Man and colleagues identified a 2-fold increase in the risk of fat necrosis (relative risk [RR], 1.94, confidence interval [CI], 1.28, 2.93) and flap loss (RR, 2.05, CI, 1.16, 3.61) in DIEP flaps compared with free TRAM flaps, whereas the risk of an abdominal bulge or hernia was approximately half (RR, 0.49, CI, 0.28, 0.86).[29] There was no difference in the risk of fat necrosis when the analysis was limited to studies using muscle-sparing free TRAM flaps (RR, 0.91, CI, 0.47, 1.78). Nahabedian and colleagues[4] studied 163 flaps in 135 patients (143 free TRAM and 20 DIEP flaps). In free TRAM flaps, the incidence of postoperative reexploration was 7.7%. Total necrosis occurred in 5 flaps (3.5%), fat necrosis was observed in 14 flaps (9.8%), an abdominal bulge developed in 8 women (6.8%), and no partial necrosis was seen. In the DIEP group, 3 flaps were reexplored (15%), total necrosis occurred in 1 flap (5%), fat necrosis developed in 2 flaps (10%), and no abdominal bulges were encountered.

SELECTION OF FLAP

The selection of flap type and design should be made based on patient weight, the amount of abdominal fat available, and breast volume requirements. In addition, the number, caliber, and location of the perforating vessels should be considered.[4] Perforator size, location, intramuscular and subcutaneous course, and association with motor nerves are significant factors that can influence operative technique, length of operation, and operative outcomes.[30] The learning curve for this procedure can be relatively steep.[31] Man and colleagues[29] state that "the most important part of that learning curve has not been the technical component of these procedures but rather the development of intraoperative decision making in choosing the appropriate technique in a given patient. The critical element of that decision is predicting high flap reliability based on anatomic findings, simultaneously limiting the potential for abdominal wall complications. Inherent in this decision is the cumulative experience of each surgeon." Kroll's[27] series demonstrated an incidence of partial flap loss of 37.5% and of fat necrosis of 62.5% in the first 8 patients, which improved to

8.7% and 17.4%, respectively, when modified selection criteria were used.

The art of this surgical procedure centers on the determination of the perforators that maximally perfuse the transferred flap while minimizing neuromuscular damage to the rectus abdominis muscle. This determination can be difficult considering the variability in the anatomy of the anterior abdominal wall vasculature. The number, location, and course of DIEPs are highly variable among patients as well as between the individual sides of the abdomen.[11,20] Proponents of the use of lateral row perforators highlight the shorter intramuscular course of these perforators, thereby facilitating shorter operative times and ease of dissection.[32] In angiographic cadaveric studies, however, lateral row perforators have vascular territories similar to that of SIEA flaps, namely, those confined to one side of the abdomen without crossing the midline.[17] Medial perforators have been demonstrated to supply a larger vascular territory compared with lateral perforators (296 cm^2 vs 196 cm^2) in an angiographic study[16] and are much more likely to perfuse across the midline, at times even into zone IV.[16,18] These considerations are important regarding volume requirements and perforator selection in unilateral cases.

The relationship of the deep inferior epigastric perforators and the motor nerves to the rectus abdominis muscle as well as the transverse distance traversed by the perforators used in the flap are also crucial to this procedure. The motor nerves to the rectus abdominis muscle enter into a nerve plexus running with the lateralmost branch of the deep inferior epigastric artery (DIEA), placing the nerves at risk when a lateral perforator is chosen.[33] The medial branches, on the other hand, are devoid of these nerve branches. The DIEA branching pattern is closely correlated with the course of the perforators.[34] A bifurcating (type II) branching pattern of the DIEA has a reduced transverse distance crossed by each perforator through the rectus abdominis muscle compared with a trifurcating (type III) branching pattern (mean, 1.4 cm vs 1.73 cm, respectively). Type I vessels are intermediate in the transverse distance each perforator travels compared with type II and III branching patterns. Another study indicates that the average perforator traverses the muscle at a distance of 1.32 cm in width, thereby requiring a sacrifice of at least that width of muscle to harvest the flap.[11] A perforator with a long intramuscular course (>4 cm) lengthens the time for operative dissection substantially, particularly when the intramuscular course occurs in a stepwise fashion.[13] All these factors should be considered when harvesting a DIEP flap. The largest perforators with the least sacrifice to the neuromuscular anatomy of the rectus abdominis muscle should be chosen.

As experience has been gained in these procedures, the importance of determining an individual's unique anatomy has become paramount. Preoperative imaging to facilitate flap harvest and determining the proposed operative plan are therefore important to expedite the procedure, reduce complications, and ease decision making, thereby decreasing surgeon stress related to the procedure. Imaging techniques can help avoid catastrophic complications caused by congenital absence or iatrogenic ligation of the deep inferior epigastric source vessels, a condition being encountered more frequently,[20,35,36] or aberrant communication of perforators with abnormal underlying source vessels.[37] The authors have encountered both of these conditions intraoperatively as well as on preoperative imaging studies (**Fig. 1**). Imaging techniques can also determine the feasibility of the procedure after previous abdominal operations, particularly after abdominal suction–assisted lipectomy or abdominoplasty (Krochmal DJ, Rebecca AM, Kalkbrenner KA, et al. Deep inferior epigastric perforator (DIEP) flap breast reconstruction after abdominal suction-assisted lipectomy, submitted for publication).[38–45]

Doppler Ultrasonography

Acoustic Doppler sonography has been used for a considerable period of time to facilitate flap harvest and to aid in preoperative flap planning.[46]

The advantages include the technique's simplicity of use, ready availability, and high sensitivity. However, this technique provides very little anatomic detail. In a study of 38 abdominally based free flaps (32 DIEP and 6 MS-TRAM flaps), Giunta and colleagues[47] reported a low false-negative rate for preoperative localization of perforators with a hand-held Doppler (14 of 127; 11%); however, the false-positive results were very high (127 perforators identified intraoperatively of the 219 marked with Doppler preoperatively; false-positive rate 42%). Doppler ultrasonography is thought to be sufficient to demonstrate an overall view of the distribution of the individual perforating vessels, and this speeds the surgical dissection and eases the intraoperative localization of the vessels.

Multidetector row computed tomography (MDCT) and computed tomographic angiography (CTA) have revolutionized anatomic imaging throughout the body. MDCT allows for rapid acquisition of a large volume of information that can be used to construct multidimensional images of small vessels. CTA has been used effectively to map the vasculature in many anatomic regions of the body, including the head and lower limbs.[48,49] The images obtained provide accurate and detailed representations of the source vessels, the perforators and associated side branches, their relationship to the muscle and fascia, and their subcutaneous branching pattern (**Fig. 2**). MDCT is touted as being significantly more accurate in localizing the site of musculocutaneous and septocutaneous perforators compared with

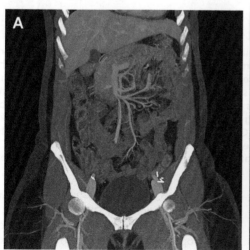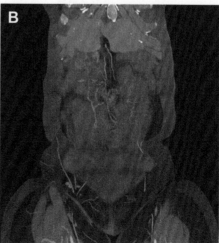

Fig. 1. (*A*) Coronal computed tomographic (CT) angiogram demonstrating iatrogenic occlusion of bilateral deep inferior epigastric systems with hemoclips from a prior gynecologic procedure. (*B*) Coronal CT angiogram of the same patient showing no filling of either deep inferior epigastric system below the umbilicus. The deep superior epigastric system and the superficial inferior epigastric veins remain patent. (*From* Casey WJ, Chew RT, Rebecca AM, et al. Advantages of preoperative computed tomography in deep inferior epigastric artery perforator flap breast reconstruction. Plast Reconstr Surg 2009;123(4):1148–55; with permission.)

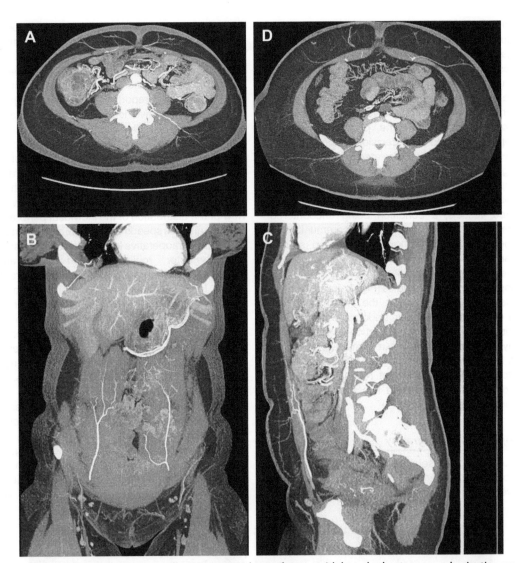

Fig. 2. (*A*) Axial CTA depicting an excellent paramuscular perforator with broad subcutaneous arborization wrapping around the medial border of the left rectus abdominis muscle. Harvest of this perforator should result in less damage to the rectus muscle compared with those seen on the right with their long transverse intramuscular course. (*B*) Coronal CTA demonstrating a type I DIEA system on the right and a type II DIEA system on the left. Identifying perforators based on a type II system tends to allow for flap harvest with less muscle damage because of their shorter intramuscular course to the underlying source vessels. (*C*) Sagittal CTA showing a musculocutaneous perforator and multiple associated side branches. Communication with the superficial inferior epigastric vein is also evident. (*D*) Axial CTA demonstrating a left lateral row perforator with an extreme lateral course. Preoperative knowledge of the subcutaneous branching pattern can assist in flap design to maximize flap perfusion and potentially minimize the risk of fat necrosis.

Doppler ultrasonography. In a study of 5 adult men, Imai and colleagues[50] detected 83 perforators originating from the deep inferior epigastric system using MDCT. Of these, only 35 perforators were identified using Doppler ultrasonography. MDCT was able to precisely localize the site of fascial penetration of the perforator, whereas Doppler ultrasonography was less accurate, with the location marked with Doppler found at an average of 7.6 mm away from the actual site based

on MDCT images (range, 0–22.5 mm). In a study of 8 patients undergoing DIEP flap surgery, Rozen and colleagues[51] compared the abilities of CTA and Doppler ultrasonography to localize and characterize the proposed perforators to use in the flap design. CTA was highly specific (100%) and more sensitive in mapping and visualizing perforators (*P* = .0078). CTA was good at identifying the SIEA system, effectively demonstrated major branches of the DIEA and perforators, and was useful in providing the images intraoperatively if needed, whereas Doppler was not. CTA was thought to be quicker to perform (15 minutes vs up to 2 hours) and removed interobserver error associated with Doppler ultrasonography. Because the clinical dissection of perforators often proved to be discordant from unidirectional Doppler flowmetry findings, Vandevoort and colleagues[13] did not use this technique for preoperative mapping of the perforators.

Duplex Ultrasonography

Duplex ultrasonography is thought to be superior to hand-held acoustic Doppler sonography in the mapping of perforator vessels. This technique combines gray-scale ultrasonography to visualize the architecture of the body part as well as color Doppler ultrasonography to estimate blood flow velocities within the vessels. This combination can assist the surgeon in locating the surface location of the proposed perforator via a simple noninvasive modality that does not require ionizing radiation or contrast material. Blondeel and colleagues[52] report a positive predictive value of almost 100% and true positive rate with the use

of duplex ultrasonography in the planning of perforator flaps. However, this study does not comment on the rate of false-negative results. Duplex ultrasonography has the disadvantage of requiring skilled technicians to complete and interpret the study, and the images are not available to the operating surgeon at the time of the procedure. CTA, on the other hand, can be read by the surgeon and provides images that can be referenced at the time of surgery (**Fig. 3**). Duplex ultrasonography also tends to have poor test-retest reliability. Other concerns pertain to the technique's inability to accurately study the branching pattern of the DIEA system, poor identification of major branches associated with the perforators, and poor visualization of the SIEA system.

Scott and colleagues[53] prospectively studied 30 flaps (4 MS-TRAM, 18 DIEP, and 8 SIEA flaps) in 22 patients. All patients underwent preoperative imaging with both CTA and duplex ultrasonography. The two largest perforators visualized with each study were chosen on both sides of the abdomen and compared based on intraoperative findings. CTA identified 83 perforators. Only 55 (66%) were demonstrated via duplex ultrasonography. Eight SIEA flaps were transferred during

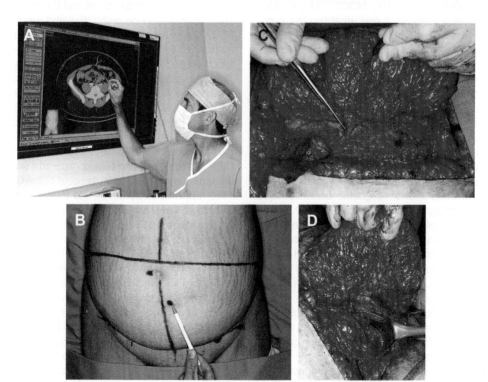

Fig. 3. (A) CTA images can be reviewed and interpreted by the operating surgeon at the time of the procedure. The images allow for precise localization of the perforators chosen in the DIEP flap design at the skin level (B) and where the perforator penetrates the anterior rectus sheath (C). (D) The multiplanar CTA images provide accurate representations of the perforators, associated side branches, and the underlying DIEA source vessels. The optimal perforators can be chosen with the least potential damage to the rectus abdominis muscle.

the study, all of which were visible with preoperative CTA. No superficial inferior epigastric systems were identified preoperatively with duplex ultrasonography. Based on the superior anatomic detail provided by CTA, the ability to characterize the SIEA system, and the significant number of clinically important perforators missed with duplex ultrasonography, the investigators conclude that CTA is a more-valuable resource for the preoperative planning of perforator flaps.

MDCT/CTA

In 2006, Masia and colleagues[54] introduced the use of MDCT for the preoperative planning of DIEP flaps. In a prospective study by Rozen and colleagues,[55] CTA was found to be highly accurate in identifying and mapping the perforators of the DIEA system. A total of 279 perforators were accurately recorded with only 1 false-positive and 1 false-negative, producing a sensitivity of 99.6% and a positive predictive value of 99.6%. All the perforators used in the flap harvest had been identified preoperatively via CTA imaging. In this study, there were no partial or total flap losses, there was no reported donor site morbidity, and there was a fat necrosis rate of 7%. MDCT/CTA provides extraordinarily high resolution, enabling the demonstration of perforators as small as 0.3 mm.[51] This high resolution is important in not only identifying the perforator itself and its communication with the underlying source vessel but also outlining its branching pattern and the linking vessels that allow communication with adjacent vascular territories to maximize the perfusion of the flap.[16] This identification and outlining becomes critical when designing the adipocutaneous flap island to minimize fat necrosis and partial flap loss. Ohjimi and colleagues[56] critically studied the vascular architecture of deep inferior epigastric–based oblique free flaps radiographically. An average of 2.1 large deep inferior epigastric perforators was included in each of 11 flaps. In 9 of the 11 flaps, the axial artery was visible. Three flaps developed partial necrosis. In 2 flaps, no axial vessels were visible, and in the third, only 1-sided distribution of the axial vessel was noted. This information further supports the idea that preoperative identification of not only the perforator itself but also its associated area of perfusion is important, which can now be defined preoperatively.

Alonso-Burgos and colleagues[57] suggested the benefits of preoperative CTA in the planning and execution of DIEP flap reconstruction early in the history of its use. In 2006, the investigators reported their experience in 6 patients. Accurate identification of the main perforators was achieved in all cases with very satisfactory concordance between CTA and the surgical findings. No unreported vessels were found. The investigators were also pleased with the characterization of the SIEA system and the fine detail provided even in the case of very small perforators. They stated that preoperative localization of adequate vessels would make the procedure easier and would decrease morbidity by preventing unnecessary perforator dissections and therefore allow the flap harvest to proceed in a faster and safer way. However, surgical outcomes and operative time were not formally studied.

To adopt CTA for routine use in perforator flap planning, its benefits must outweigh its disadvantages and risks. CTA requires the infusion of intravenous contrast. As such, those with contrast or iodine allergies or those with renal impairment have contraindications for the use of CTA. CTA also exposes the patient to ionizing radiation. Recent literature cautions against the rising number of computed tomography (CT) scans performed because of the associated radiation exposure.[58] With the use of MDCT, the effective dose of radiation is relatively low. This dose has been reported to be between 4.8 and 6 mSv, which is less than that of a conventional abdominal CT scan.[30,59,60] The cost can also be prohibitive and ranges from ¥1000 (approximately $150)[59] to £350 (approximately $556)[61] to $1734 (United States in 2008) for combined hospital and professional charges.[60] The estimated savings due to reduced operative times alone has been quoted as £1750 (approximately $2779) by expediting flap harvest times based on the information that CTA provides.[62] Uppal and colleagues[61] reported a mean reduction in the operative time of 76 minutes for unilateral DIEP flap transfer using CTA compared with duplex ultrasonography. Although the cost of the CTA was £176 (approximately $275), the 21% reduction in operative time resulted in a savings of £471 (approximately $732) from anesthesia and facility costs alone. The investigators then made reference to a study by Jenkins and Baker,[63] pointing out that prolonged operative time can increase postoperative recovery and may increase complications such as atelectasis and deep vein thrombosis. Reduction in operative time for these intricate procedures may minimize the risk of these complications. It is for these reasons that detailed outcome studies are important to validate the use of CTA in the planning of perforator flaps.

MDCT/CTA Operative Time

One of the primary advantages of using CTA in the preoperative planning of perforator flaps centers around shortening the learning curve for the procedure and reducing operative time to harvest and transfer the flap. CTA may flatten the learning curve and shorten the time to proficiency for less-experienced surgeons. This may limit flap-specific complications (partial/complete flap loss, fat necrosis, or anastomotic complications) and donor site complications (abdominal bulges, hernias, abdominal weakness, or abdominal wounds) early in a surgeon's experience with perforator flaps. Reducing operative time directly reduces the cost of the procedure by decreasing anesthesia and facility costs. Reducing flap-specific and donor site complications can also reduce costs by reducing hospital length of stay, secondary procedures, and the supplies required to address a complication.

Casey and colleagues[36] demonstrated a reduction in operative time in unilateral DIEP flap transfer from 459 minutes to 370 minutes following the routine use of CTA compared with hand-held Doppler interrogation alone. In bilateral cases, operative times were reduced from 657 minutes to 515 minutes. The decreased operative time in this retrospectively designed study was thought to be because of a more-directed dissection to the dominant perforator with the most direct intramuscular course as compared with a blind exploration of the anterior abdominal wall when a hand-held Doppler was used alone. A correlation between surgeon experience and operative time was also performed in this study. With the use of CTA, the surgeon with the least experience was quickly able to match the operative times of the most senior surgeon with similar overall flap and donor site complication rates. This information supports the benefits of CTA in shortening the learning curve for DIEP flap reconstruction.

Uppal and colleagues[61] prospectively studied 26 patients scheduled to undergo perforator flap breast reconstruction (unilateral/bilateral DIEP, superior gluteal artery perforator [SGAP] flaps). Mean operative times for unilateral DIEP, bilateral DIEP, and SGAP flap reconstruction were 4 hours and 49 minutes, 7 hours and 23 minutes, and 4 hours and 56 minutes, respectively. Compared with 15 unilateral DIEP duplex controls, operative time was shorter by 1 hour and 16 minutes (21% reduction) in the CTA group. Minqiang and colleagues[59] specifically studied the time required to harvest a DIEP flap. Between December 2006 and May 2008, 22 consecutive patients who underwent CTA before DIEP breast reconstruction were compared with 22 previous patients who did not undergo CTA. The time required to harvest a DIEP flap was 2.8 ± 0.2 hours in the CTA group compared with 4.4 ± 0.2 hours in the control group (no CTA).

Smit and colleagues[62] performed a chart review of 138 DIEP breast reconstructions. Of these, 70 were performed after preoperative CTA and were compared with 68 flap reconstructions that were performed the previous year using Doppler examination alone. Operative time in the CTA group was 264 minutes compared with 354 minutes in the Doppler control group. Rozen and colleagues[64] prospectively studied 40 patients who underwent breast reconstruction after CTA between March 2006 and November 2007. These patients were compared with 48 patients who had previously undergone breast reconstruction without CTA. CTA resulted in a reduction in operative time by 77 minutes and was noted to be even more beneficial in bilateral cases. This study also included a psychometric assessment of operative stress for the operating surgeon during perforator dissection with and without the use of CTA. A statistically significant reduction of 41% in the mean stress level experienced by the operating surgeon was encountered with the use of CTA. Masia and colleagues[65] reported on 90 patients and found an average operating time savings of 1 hour and 40 minutes when CTA was used preoperatively. In a follow-up study, Masia and colleagues[66] confirmed these findings in 357 patients, showing a significant decrease in the time needed for DIEP flap harvest from 3 hours and 20 minutes to 1 hour and 40 minutes.

Flap-related Complications

CTA has the theoretical advantage of being able to preoperatively localize the dominant perforators based on their relative size and branching patterns that adequately supply a flap. This ability is particularly important in unilateral cases. In bilateral cases, the perforators can be approached both laterally as well as medially once the 2 sides of the abdominal skin is divided in the midline. In unilateral cases, however, it can be difficult to visualize medial row perforators without sacrificing their lateral counterparts. Without this information preoperatively, a truly dominant lateral perforator may be sacrificed to visualize what are later found to be less-suitable medial row vessels. In a collective experience of 600 flaps over a span of 12 months, Massey and colleagues[1] report a total flap failure rate of 1%. These excellent results highlight that CTA is unlikely to result in a significant improvement in the rate of total flap loss. This technique is likely to have more of an effect on the rate of fat necrosis and partial flap loss by maximizing the perfusion of the distal segments of the flap by designing the flap around the best perforasome.[18]

Rozen and colleagues[67] evaluated 75 patients prospectively to highlight the utility of CTA. In this series, there was a flap survival of 100% with no partial or complete flap losses. In 3 cases, CTA dictated whether an operation was appropriate at all. Seven unique cases were presented to demonstrate the importance of CTA, which included cases in which previous surgery altered or disrupted the vascular anatomy; cases in which small perforators were seen, therefore dictating that an MS-TRAM should be performed; a case in which a DIEP flap could be harvested despite a ventral hernia; and cases in which CTA identified comorbid conditions that influenced the decision to proceed. In 15 cases (20%), the expected operation was directly changed because of the imaging results. Minqiang and colleagues[59] experienced an incidence of 22.7% of preoperative flap redesign based on CTA findings. The intraoperative plan remained the same in all patients in the CTA group, whereas the intraoperative plan changed in 13.6% in those who did not have a preoperative CTA. There was 1 case of partial flap loss in the CTA group, and 1 complete loss and 2 partial flap losses in the control group.

In a study of 287 DIEP flap breast reconstructions, Casey and colleagues[36] reported a fat necrosis rate of 10.9% in procedures performed after CTA. Although this rate was better than the 13.4% experienced in cases performed with Doppler examination alone, this did not reach statistical significance. The incidence of anastomotic complications and total flap loss was also similar between the CTA and Doppler groups (6.9% vs 8.1% and 2% vs 3.8%, respectively). Uppal and colleagues[61] evaluated 17 unilateral and 12 bilateral DIEP flap reconstructions after CTA. Fat necrosis was noted in 1 bilateral case and in none of the unilateral cases. Only 1 postoperative reexploration was necessary in 1 of the bilateral cases. Smit and colleagues[62] identified fewer complications in a CTA group compared with the non-CTA control group (20% vs 25%). The CTA group had 6 infections, 4 hematomas, 2 superficial necroses, 2 seromas, and 2 anastomotic complications. The control group included 6 infections, 4 hematomas, 6 superficial necroses, and 6 anastomotic complications. All flap reconstructions were successful in the CTA group, whereas 1 flap reconstruction failed and partial necrosis occurred in 3 flaps in the control group.

In a study by Rozen and colleagues[64] of 40 patients following CTA and 48 prior patients without CTA, no partial flap losses were encountered in the CTA group, whereas 5 occurred in the control group. Fat necrosis was also less common in the CTA group (3/40, 7.5% vs 8/48,

16.7%). No complete flap losses occurred in either group. In the largest study to date, Masia[66] prospectively evaluated 357 patients scheduled for DIEP flap breast reconstruction. Total flap loss was reduced from 4% to 1% after the introduction of CTA. In addition, partial flap loss greater than 20% and partial flap loss less than 20% were reduced from 6% to 2% and 6% to 0%, respectively.

Donor Site Complications

Another advantage of CTA lies in its ability to identify a suitable perforator with an intramuscular course, which on harvesting minimizes the neuromuscular damage to the rectus abdominis muscle. Finding a dominant medial row perforator with a paramuscular or paraneural anatomic course can be ideal, allowing for a more simplified harvest and minimal trauma to the rectus abdominis muscle.[15,33] This was found to occur in 11% of cases in the largest series of DIEP flap reconstructions after CTA to date.[66] If this anatomic configuration does not exist, then CTA can demonstrate a perforator with the shortest transverse intramuscular course with the fewest associated side branches. By limiting the division of rectus muscle fibers and preserving the motor nerves, complications such as bulges, hernias, and abdominal weakness can be minimized. CTA can potentially increase a surgeon's comfort in the inclusion of less perforators in the flap design, thereby limiting the division of intervening muscle fibers between neighboring vessels.

Casey and colleagues[36] demonstrated a significant reduction in the number of incorporated perforators in DIEP flap design after the introduction of preoperative CTA perforator mapping. The incidence of postoperative abdominal bulges dropped precipitously once a CTA protocol was instituted. Using hand-held Doppler alone, the rate of abdominal bulges after DIEP flap transfer was 9.1%. After CTA, this rate dropped to 1% with similar abdominal closure techniques. When the analysis was limited to a single surgeon, the incidence of postoperative abdominal wound complications was also significantly reduced in the CTA group compared with the group that used hand-held Doppler only (3/41, 7% vs 12/41, 29%, respectively). In Rozen and colleagues'[64] prospective study of 104 DIEP flaps in 88 patients (40 with CTA, 48 without CTA), a significant reduction in donor site morbidity was encountered in the CTA group (0/40, 0% vs 7/48, 14.6%). Abdominal bulges were reduced from 2.1% to 0%, and abdominal hernias dropped from 12.5% to 0%.

Future Modalities

CTA has become an invaluable tool in the preoperative planning of perforator flaps. At present, 7 of 10 investigators in a large series recently published use some form of preoperative imaging routinely for every case of perforator flap breast reconstruction.[1] As technology advances, our search for less invasive means to provide more detailed and accurate information continues. Virtual reality software can improve the accuracy of perforator localization.[68,69] Magnetic resonance angiography has the benefit of requiring no iodinated intravenous contrast material and does not subject the patient to ionizing radiation. Preliminary experience with this technique is encouraging[70–72]; however, this study is more expensive, less reproducible, and not as good at providing fine anatomic detail of smaller perforators compared with CTA at present. Although these modalities have shown promise, at present, CTA remains the gold standard for perforator mapping. All these imaging techniques provide important information to the operating surgeon regarding the perforators; however, they do not provide all the information needed to complete the procedure. Although the general relationships regarding the DIEA branches, perforators, and the motor nerves to the rectus abdominis muscle have been described,[33] the actual association between individual nerves and vessels in any given patient cannot yet be determined based on current imaging techniques. These techniques also fail to account for physiologic changes related to blood flow and perfusion. These studies are meant as an adjunct, not a replacement for surgical judgment.

Conclusions for Autologous Breast Reconstruction

The lower abdomen has become the preferred donor site for autologous breast reconstruction. Significant variability in the anatomy of the deep inferior epigastric source vessels and their associated perforators has made preoperative imaging for perforator mapping and planning desirable. CTA has emerged as the gold standard for this purpose. CTA can accurately select the optimal perforators to maximize flap perfusion while minimizing donor site morbidity related to neuromuscular damage to the rectus abdominis muscle. The information allows a more directed dissection to the dominant perforators that have the most direct course through or around the rectus abdominis muscle to the underlying deep inferior epigastric pedicle. Preoperative imaging with CTA has been demonstrated to expedite flap harvest. This

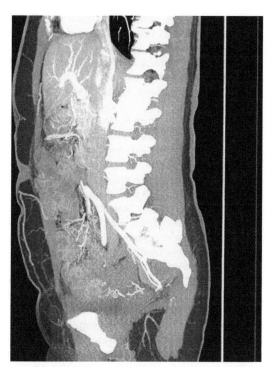

Fig. 4. Sagittal CTA showing immediate communication of a sizable periumbilical perforator with the superficial inferior epigastric vein. Recent evidence shows selection of perforators with anastomoses between the superficial and deep systems can minimize flap-related complications.

imaging decreases operative time and associated costs, reduces flap-specific complications (particularly fat necrosis and partial flap loss), and helps minimize donor site problems such as bulges and hernias. Although arterial inflow in perforator flaps is important, venous outflow issues are reported to be more critical.[61,73] Improved spatial resolution with current imaging techniques allows for better anatomic detail of the relationship between neighboring perforators and the communication between the superficial and deep systems (**Fig. 4**). This information is now being used to minimize flap complications and predict a successful outcome.[74] CTA is currently the imaging modality of choice for preoperative perforator mapping; however, many other options are available, each offering certain advantages.

REFERENCES

1. Massey MF, Spiegel AJ, Levine JL, et al. Perforator flaps: recent experience, current trends, and future directions based on 3974 microsurgical breast reconstructions. Plast Reconstr Surg 2009;124(3): 737–51.

2. Hartrampf CR Jr, Scheflan M, Black PW. Breast reconstruction with a transverse abdominal island flap. Plast Reconstr Surg 1982;69:216–25.

3. Watterson PA, Bostwick J III, Hester R Jr, et al. TRAM flap anatomy correlated with a 10-year clinical experience with 556 patients. Plast Reconstr Surg 1995; 95(7):1185–94.

4. Nahabedian MY, Momen B, Galdino G, et al. Breast reconstruction with the TRAM or DIEP flap: patient selection, choice of flap, and outcome. Plast Reconstr Surg 2002;110(2):466–75.

5. Gill PS, Hunt JP, Guerra AB, et al. A 10-year retrospective review of 758 DIEP flaps for breast reconstruction. Plast Reconstr Surg 2004;113(4):1153–60.

6. Hamdi M, Weiler-Mithoff EM, Webster MH. Deep inferior epigastric perforator flap in breast reconstruction: experience with the first 50 flaps. Plast Reconstr Surg 1999;103:86–95.

7. Blondeel PN. One hundred free DIEP flap breast reconstructions: a personal experience. Br J Plast Surg 1999;52:104–11.

8. Bonde CT, Christensen DE, Elberg JJ. Ten years' experience of free flaps for breast reconstruction in a Danish microsurgical centre: an audit. Scand J Plast Reconstr Surg Hand Surg 2006;40:8–12.

9. Boyd JB, Taylor GI, Corlett R. The vascular territories of the superior epigastric and the deep inferior epigastric systems. Plast Reconstr Surg 1984; 73(1):1–14.

10. Moon HK, Taylor GI. The vascular anatomy of rectus abdominis musculocutaneous flaps based on the deep superior epigastric system. Plast Reconstr Surg 1988;82:815–32.

11. Rozen WM, Ashton MW, Pan WR, et al. Raising perforator flaps for breast reconstruction: the intramuscular anatomy of the deep inferior epigastric artery. Plast Reconstr Surg 2007;120(6):1443–9.

12. El-Mrakby HH, Milner RH. The vascular anatomy of the lower anterior abdominal wall: a microdissection study on the deep inferior epigastric vessels and the perforator branches. Plast Reconstr Surg 2002; 109(2):539–47.

13. Vandevoort M, Vranckx JJ, Fabre G. Perforator topography of the deep inferior epigastric perforator flap in 100 cases of breast reconstruction. Plast Reconstr Surg 2002;109(6):1912–8.

14. Saint-Cyr M, Schaverien M, Arbique G, et al. Three- and four-dimensional computed tomographic angiography and venography for the investigation of the vascular anatomy and perfusion of perforator flaps. Plast Reconstr Surg 2008;121(3):772–80.

15. Gravvanis A, Dionyssiou DD, Chandrasekharan L, et al. Paramuscular and paraneural perforators in DIEAP flaps: radiographic findings and clinical application. Ann Plast Surg 2009;63(6):610–5.

16. Wong C, Saint-Cyr M, Mojallal A, et al. Perforasomes of the DIEP flap: vascular anatomy of the lateral versus medial row perforators and clinical implications. Plast Reconstr Surg 2010;125(3):772–82.

17. Wong C, Saint-Cyr M, Arbique G, et al. Three- and four-dimensional computed tomography angiographic studies of commonly used abdominal flaps in breast reconstruction. Plast Reconstr Surg 2009; 124(1):18–27.

18. Rozen WM, Ashton MW, Le Roux CM, et al. The perforator angiosome: a new concept in the design of deep inferior epigastric artery perforator flaps for breast reconstruction. Microsurgery 2009;10: 1–7.

19. Rozen WM, Ashton MW, Taylor GI. Reviewing the vascular supply of the anterior abdominal wall: redefining anatomy for increasingly refined surgery. Clin Anat 2008;21:89–98.

20. Rozen WM, Ashton MW, Grinsell D. The branching pattern of the deep inferior epigastric artery revisited in-vivo: a new classification based on CT angiography. Clin Anat 2010;23:87–92.

21. Fujino T. Contribution of the axial and perforator vasculature to circulation in flaps. Plast Reconstr Surg 1967;39(2):125–37.

22. Taylor GI, Palmer JH. The vascular territories (angiosomes) of the body: experimental study and clinical applications. Br J Plast Surg 1987;40(2):113–41.

23. Kroll SS, Rosenfield L. Perforator-based flaps for low posterior midline defects. Plast Reconstr Surg 1988; 81(4):561–6.

24. Koshima I, Soeda S. Inferior epigastric artery skin flap without rectus abdominis muscle. Br J Plast Surg 1989;42(6):645–8.

25. Allen RJ, Treece P. Deep inferior epigastric perforator flap for breast reconstruction. Ann Plast Surg 1994;32:32–8.

26. Spiegel AJ, Khan FN. An intraoperative algorithm for use of the SIEA flap for breast reconstruction. Plast Reconstr Surg 2007;120:1450–9.

27. Kroll SS. Fat necrosis in free transverse rectus abdominis myocutaneous and deep inferior epigastric perforator flaps. Plast Reconstr Surg 2000;106(3): 576–83.

28. Wu LC, Bajaj A, Chang DW, et al. Comparison of donor-site morbidity of SIEA, DIEP, and muscle-sparing TRAM flaps for breast reconstruction. Plast Reconstr Surg 2008;122(3):702–9.

29. Man LX, Selber JC, Serletti JM. Abdominal wall following free TRAM or DIEP flap reconstruction: a meta-analysis and critical review. Plast Reconstr Surg 2009;124(3):752–64.

30. Rozen WM, Ashton MW. Improving outcomes in autologous breast reconstruction. Aesthetic Plast Surg 2009;33:327–35.

31. Busic V, Das-Gupta R, Mesic H, et al. The deep inferior epigastric perforator flap for breast reconstruction, the learning curve explored. J Plast Reconstr Aesthet Surg 2006;59:580–4.

32. Munhoz AM, Ishida LH, Sturtz GP, et al. Importance of lateral row perforator vessels in deep inferior epigastric perforator flap harvesting. Plast Reconstr Surg 2004;113(2):517–24.

33. Rozen WM, Ashton MW, Murray AC, et al. Avoiding denervation of rectus abdominis in DIEP flap harvest: the importance of medial row perforators. Plast Reconstr Surg 2008;122(3):710–6.

34. Rozen WM, Palmer KP, Suami H, et al. The DIEA branching pattern and its relationship to perforators: the importance of preoperative computed tomographic angiography for DIEA perforator flaps. Plast Reconstr Surg 2008;121(2):367–73.

35. Chubb D, Rozen WM, Ashton MW. Complete absence of the deep inferior epigastric artery: an increasingly detected anomaly detected with the use of advanced imaging technologies. J Reconstr Microsurg 2010;26(3):209–10.

36. Casey WJ III, Chew RT, Rebecca AM, et al. Advantages of preoperative computed tomography in deep inferior epigastric artery perforator flap breast reconstruction. Plast Reconstr Surg 2009;123(4): 1148–55.

37. Whitaker IS, Rozen WM, Smit JM, et al. Peritoneocutaneous perforators in deep inferior epigastric perforator flaps: a cadaveric dissection and computed tomographic angiography study. Microsurgery 2009;29:124–7.

38. Salgarello M, Barone-Adesi L, Cina AL, et al. The effect of liposuction on inferior epigastric perforator vessels: a prospective study with color Doppler sonography. Ann Plast Surg 2005;55:346–51.

39. Ribuffo D, Marcellino M, Barnett GR, et al. Breast reconstruction with abdominal flaps after abdominoplasties. Plast Reconstr Surg 2001;108:1604–8.

40. Karanas Y, Santoro T, DaLio A, et al. Free TRAM flap reconstruction after abdominal liposuction. Plast Reconstr Surg 2003;112:1851–4.

41. Godfrey PM, Godfrey NV. Transverse rectus abdominis musculocutaneous flaps after liposuction of the abdomen. Ann Plast Surg 1994;33:209–10.

42. May J, Silverman R, Kaufman J. Flap perfusion mapping: TRAM flap after abdominal suction-assisted lipectomy. Plast Reconstr Surg 1999;104(7): 2278–81.

43. Hess CL, Gartside RL, Ganz JC. TRAM reconstruction after abdominal liposuction. Ann Plast Surg 2004;53(2):166–9.

44. De Frene B, Van Landuyt K, Hamdi M, et al. Free DIEAP and SGAP flap breast reconstruction after abdominal/gluteal liposuction. J Plast Reconstr Aesthet Surg 2006;59:1031–6.

45. Kim J, Chang D, Temple C, et al. Free transverse rectus abdominis musculocutaneous flap reconstruction in patients with prior abdominal suction-assisted lipectomy. Plast Reconstr Surg 2004; 113(3):28–31.

46. Taylor GI, Doyle M, McCarten G. The Doppler probe for planning flaps: anatomical study and clinical applications. Br J Plast Surg 1990;43(1):1–16.

47. Giunta RE, Geisweld A, Feller AM. The value of preoperative Doppler sonography for planning free perforator flaps. Plast Reconstr Surg 2000;105(7): 2381–6.

48. Bluemke DA, Chambers TP. Spiral CT angiography: an alternative to conventional angiography. Radiology 1995;195(2):317–9.

49. Rieker O, Duber C, Schmiedt W, et al. Prospective comparison of CT angiography of the legs with intra-arterial digital subtraction angiography. Am J Roentgenol 1996;166(2):269–76.

50. Imai R, Matsumura H, Tanaka K, et al. Comparison of Doppler sonography and multidetector-row computed tomography in the imaging findings of the deep inferior epigastric perforator artery. Ann Plast Surg 2008;61(1):94–8.

51. Rozen WM, Phillips TJ, Ashton MW, et al. Preoperative imaging for DIEA perforator flaps: a comparative study of computed tomographic angiography and Doppler ultrasound. Plast Reconstr Surg 2007; 121(1):9–16.

52. Blondeel P, Beyens G, Verhaeghe R, et al. Doppler flowmetry in the planning of perforator flaps. Br J Plast Surg 1998;51:202–9.

53. Scott JR, Liu D, Said H, et al. Computed tomographic angiography in planning abdomen-based microsurgical breast reconstruction: a comparison with color duplex ultrasound. Plast Reconstr Surg 2010;125(2):446–53.

54. Masia J, Clavero JA, Larranaga JR, et al. Multidetector-row computed tomography in the planning of abdominal perforator flaps. J Plast Reconstr Aesthet Surg 2006;59:594–9.

55. Rozen WM, Ashton MW, Stella DL, et al. The accuracy of computed tomographic angiography for mapping the perforators of the deep inferior epigastric artery: a blinded, prospective cohort study. Plast Reconstr Surg 2008;122(4):1003–9.

56. Ohjimi H, Era K, Tanahashi S, et al. Ex vivo intraoperative angiography for rectus abdominis musculocutaneous free flaps. Plast Reconstr Surg 2002;109(7): 2247–56.

57. Alonso-Burgos A, Garcia-Tutor E, Bastarrika G, et al. Preoperative planning of deep inferior epigastric artery perforator flap reconstruction with multi-slice-CT angiography: imaging findings and initial experience. J Plast Reconstr Aesthet Surg 2006; 59:585–93.

58. Brenner DJ, Hall EJ. Computed tomography: an increasing source of radiation exposure. N Engl J Med 2007;357:2277–84.

59. Minqiang X, Lanhua M, Jie L, et al. The value of multidetector-row CT angiography for pre-operative planning of breast reconstruction with deep inferior

epigastric arterial perforator flaps. Br J Radiol 2010; 83:40–3.

60. Mathes DW, Neligan PC. Current techniques in preoperative imaging for abdomen-based perforator flap microsurgical breast reconstruction. J Reconstr Microsurg 2010;26(1):3–10.

61. Uppal RS, Casaer B, Van Landuyt K, et al. The efficacy of preoperative mapping of perforators in reducing operative times and complications in perforator flap breast reconstruction. J Plast Reconstr Aesthet Surg 2009;62:859–64.

62. Smit JM, Dimopoulou A, Liss AG, et al. Preoperative CT angiography reduces surgery time in perforator flap reconstruction. J Plast Reconstr Aesthet Surg 2009;62:1112–7.

63. Jenkins K, Baker AB. Consent and anaesthetic risk. Anaesthesia 2003;58:962–84.

64. Rozen WM, Anavekar NS, Ashton MW, et al. Does the preoperative imaging of perforators with CT angiography improve outcomes in breast reconstruction? Microsurgery 2008;28:516–23.

65. Masia J, Larranaga J, Clavero JA, et al. The value of the multidetector row computed tomography for the preoperative planning of deep inferior epigastric artery perforator flap: our experience in 162 cases. Ann Plast Surg 2008;60:29–36.

66. Masia J, Kosutic D, Clavero JA, et al. Preoperative computed tomographic angiogram for deep inferior epigastric artery perforator flap breast reconstruction. J Reconstr Microsurg 2010;26(1):21–8.

67. Rozen WM, Ashton MW, Grinsell D, et al. Establishing the case for CT angiography in the preoperative imaging of abdominal wall perforators. Microsurgery 2008;28:306–13.

68. Pacifico MD, See MS, Cavale N, et al. Preoperative planning for DIEP breast reconstruction: early experience of the use of computerized tomography angiography with VoNavix 3D software for perforator navigation. J Plast Reconstr Aesthet Surg 2009;62: 1464–9.

69. Gacto-Sanchez P, Sicilia-Castro D, Gomez-Cia T, et al. Use of a three-dimensional virtual reality model for preoperative imaging in DIEP flap breast reconstruction. J Surg Res 2010;162(1):140–7.

70. Alonso-Burgos A, Garcia-Tutor E, Bastarrika G, et al. Preoperative planning of DIEP and SGAP flaps: preliminary experience with magnetic resonance angiography using 3-tesla equipment and blood-pool contrast medium. J Plast Reconstr Aesthet Surg 2010;63:298–304.

71. Neil-Dwyer JG, Ludman CN, Schaverien M, et al. Magnetic resonance angiography in preoperative planning of deep inferior epigastric artery perforator flaps. J Plast Reconstr Aesthet Surg 2009;62:1661–5.

72. Rozen WM, Stella DL, Bowden J, et al. Advances in the pre-operative planning of deep inferior epigastric artery perforator flaps: magnetic resonance angiography. Microsurgery 2009;29:119–23.

73. Blondeel PN, Arnstein M, Verstraete K, et al. Venous congestion and blood flow in free transverse rectus abdominis myocutaneous and deep inferior epigastric perforator flaps. Plast Reconstr Surg 2000;106: 1295–9.

74. Schaverien MV, Ludman CN, Neil-Dwyer J, et al. Relationship between venous congestion and intra-flap venous anatomy in DIEP flaps using contrast-enhanced magnetic resonance angiography. Plast Reconstr Surg 2010;126(2):385–92.

Noncontrast Magnetic Resonance Imaging for Preoperative Perforator Mapping

Jaume Masia, MD, PhD[a],*, Carmen Navarro, MD[a],
Juan A. Clavero, MD, PhD[b], Xavier Alomar, MD, PhD[b]

KEYWORDS

- MRI • MDCT • Perforator mapping • DIEP flap
- Breast reconstruction • AngioCT

The deep inferior epigastric artery perforator (DIEP) flap has gained immense popularity in breast reconstruction since its introduction in the 1990s.[1-3] It provides fat and skin with characteristics that are similar to those of the normal breast and spares the rectus abdominis muscle or fascia, thereby minimizing donor site morbidity.[4] One of the key points in breast reconstruction with DIEP flap is choosing the best supplying perforator[5] and several factors should be kept in mind when doing so. The ideal perforator vessel should have a large caliber, a short intramuscular course, the easiest dissection, a suitable location within the flap, and subcutaneous branching with intraflap axiality. In our experience, after performing more than 600 DIEP flaps, we have identified perforator vessels with a totally extramuscular course in 12% of cases. These extramuscular vessels initially follow a retromuscular plane before piercing the muscular fascia in the exact abdominal midline. They are thus paramuscular perforator vessels rather than musculocutaneous perforator vessels. We consider these vessels to be ideal because their course facilitates dissection.[6]

Perforator vessels arising from the deep inferior epigastric system are anatomically highly variable in number, location, caliber, and relationships with surrounding structures[7,8] In view of this variability, is it valuable to have a reliable method that accurately identifies and locates the dominant perforator before surgery.[5,9] Precise imaging can help to select the best hemiabdomen to raise, to differentiate between superficial and deep epigastric vessels and to combine 2 or more perforator vessels when there is no dominant vessel. A precise image allows planning of the operative technique, reduction of operating time, and improvement in operative outcomes.[10] Using preoperative imaging techniques to study the epigastric vessels, we have decreased the number of postoperative complications.[11]

METHODS MOST WIDELY USED AT PRESENT FOR THE PREOPERATIVE STUDY OF ABDOMINAL PERFORATING VESSELS

Several techniques are available for the preoperative mapping of abdominal perforating vessels: handheld Doppler ultrasound, color Doppler imaging, computed tomography-angiography (CTA), and, more recently, magnetic resonance imaging (MRI).

The handheld Doppler ultrasound has been in use since the early days of microsurgery. This easy-to-use, inexpensive technique is performed by surgeons to locate the perforating arteries before perforator flap elevation, and it is the method most commonly used to locate an

The authors have no financial interests in the devices mentioned in the text.
[a] Plastic Surgery Department, Hospital de la Santa Creu i Sant Pau (Universidad Autónoma de Barcelona), Sant Antoni Maria Claret 167, Barcelona 08025, Spain
[b] Radiology Department, Clínica Creu Blanca, Reina Elisenda de Montcada 17, Barcelona 08034, Spain
* Corresponding author.
E-mail address: jmasia@santpau.cat

Clin Plastic Surg 38 (2011) 253–261
doi:10.1016/j.cps.2011.03.004
0094-1298/11/$ – see front matter © 2011 Published by Elsevier Inc.

individual vessel before surgery.[12,13] However, correlation between the audible volume of the signal and the diameter of the perforator vessel is poor and often imprecise.[9,12] It offers only a limited amount of information and cannot distinguish perforator vessels from main axial vessels. It does not provide any data on the course of the perforator vessel because the information is given as an acoustic signal. The number of false positives is high, reaching 47% in one series.[9] The value of Doppler sonography in this setting is therefore questionable. Doppler sonography may also be too sensitive because even minuscule vessels that are not large enough to support a perforator flap can be selected for abdominal perforator surgery. Despite these drawbacks, handheld Doppler ultrasound remains useful in our daily practice and helps us to assess the situation and the course of the superficial epigastric vessels.

Color Doppler imaging provides more information than Doppler sonography. It is a highly reliable technique to identify and locate the dominant perforator vessel.[14] It provides a good evaluation of the main axial vessels and their perforator vessels. Moreover, the caliber and hemodynamic characteristics of the perforator vessels can be observed directly on color Doppler imaging. It provides information about blood flow direction, pattern, and velocity. The high sensitivity and the 100% predictive value of this technique have made it a good diagnostic tool in the planning of DIEP flaps.[12] However, color Doppler imaging also has some limitations; it is time consuming for the radiologist to perform and patients are often uncomfortable because they must remain in the same position for nearly 1 hour. In addition, it requires the presence of highly skilled sonographers with knowledge of perforator flap surgery, and its results are technician dependent. In addition, color Doppler imaging does not provide anatomic images that show the surgeon the anatomic relationship between the deep inferior epigastric artery and its perforator branches and other structures along its route. These important limitations have contributed to its disuse in microsurgical units.

Since 2003, the multidetector-row computed tomography (MDCT) scan has proved to be highly reliable in preoperative planning of abdominal free flap breast reconstruction[15-20] and has shown excellent results, significantly reducing operative time and complications. Unlike the handheld Doppler and colored duplex-Doppler ultrasound, it provides anatomic images that are easy to interpret and offers information on the caliber, location, and course of any perforating vessel.[21] With the recent development of MDCT, a considerable number of thin-sliced computed tomography (CT) images are obtained in a short time. Intravenous contrast medium can be injected at high velocities, and excellent images of the vasculature are obtained. The increased spatial resolution offered by MDCT allows highly accurate multiplanar and 3D reconstructed images to be obtained.[16] Moreover, this technique is easily reproducible and fast to perform, thereby minimizing patient discomfort and health care costs compared with the color Doppler technique. In addition, it provides unique and valuable information for surgical planning. The main drawbacks of CT are unnecessary radiation to the patient (effective dose is 5.6 mSv, similar to conventional abdominal CT scan[11,22]) and potential systemic allergic reactions to the intravenous contrast medium.[23,24]

NONCONTRAST MRI

To overcome the limitation of radiation with the MDCT technique, in 2005 we began to investigate the possibility of using MRI for abdominal perforator mapping. In the following 3 years we worked with different kinds of MRI technologies, but all of them needed a contrast injection to obtain a good quality image of the perforator vessels. These MRI techniques allowed us to visualize perforator vessels with the same reliability as MDCT. A comparative study with 30 patients showed that there were no false positives. However, we found that the technique had several drawbacks. First, intravenous contrast was still necessary to obtain adequate quality images. Second, the image resolution did not allow precise analysis of the perforators' intramuscular course and its anatomic relationships. In addition, the 3D image reconstruction was not as accurate as with MDCT. Although this is not essential for surgery, such pictures can be useful for teaching purposes. Other disadvantages were the possible claustrophobic feeling for the patients and that they had to lie face down to avoid respiratory movement.

However, we decided continue, and 1 year later we began to study the usefulness of 3-Tesla (T) MRI. This technique provided high-resolution images that allowed us to study the intramuscular and subfascial course of the perforating vessels. We acquired the images in less time, and contrast visibility with the same dose of gadolinium was better. Other investigators have since stressed the value of this technique.[25] However, this technology is expensive and not available at all centers. In addition, intravenous contrast administration is still required.

During our investigation at this time our attention was drawn to methods being used for the study of renal tumors with noncontrast MRI. This technique allowed good visualization of the vessels and we began to consider the possibility of using the same sequence for preoperative perforator mapping of the abdominal wall in female patients undergoing breast reconstruction with DIEP flap after mastectomy. In 2007, we found a new 1.5-T MRI acquisition sequence that provided specific vascular imaging without using contrast material.

At first, we used a 1.5-T magnetic resonance (MR) system (Excelart Vantage; Toshiba Medical Systems, Tokyo, Japan) equipped with a pair of 4-by-4 phased array coils. We used a respiratory-triggered, 3D true, steady-state, free-precession (SSFP) imaging sequence with time spatial inversion pulse (T-SLIP). We performed this in anterior coronal and axial planes using the following parameters: repetition time (TR)/echo time (TE)/facet angle (FA), 5.2 milliseconds/2.6 milliseconds/120°; slice thickness, 1.5 mm for coronal and 5 mm for axial planes; slice number, 40 to 50, no gap; field of view, 400×350 mm, matrix 256×256; number of acquisitions, 1. The acquisition time ranged from 20 to 30 minutes.

Despite the correct localization of the dominant perforator in all patients, in some cases we noted a low definition of the perforator course inside the muscle, which meant that some critical information for an effective perforator mapping was lost compared with MDCT.

We then started working with Toshiba engineers in an attempt to improve the image acquisition sequence. We decided to switch to a new MR angiography technique called fresh blood imaging

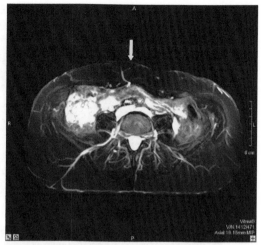

Fig. 2. Axial magnetic resonance image of the chosen perforator with its branching to both the ipsilateral and contralateral sides. The yellow arrow indicates the point at which the perforator arises from the muscle.

(FBI) with a Toshiba ZGV Vantage ATLAS 1.5-T, ultrashort-bore body MR system (Toshiba Medical Systems, Tokyo, Japan). This technique provided accurate location of the dominant perforator, good definition of its intramuscular course and excellent evaluation of the superficial inferior epigastric system. We were also able to define the perforator branching within the subcutaneous abdominal tissue and evaluate the vascular connections between the superficial and the deep inferior epigastric vessels (**Figs. 1–3**).

With the noncontrast SSFP imaging sequence 1.5-T MRI technique, we found 42% insufficiency

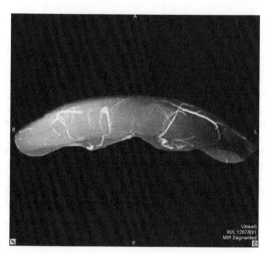

Fig. 1. Sagittal magnetic resonance image. Several perforators and their branching to the ipsilateral side can be seen.

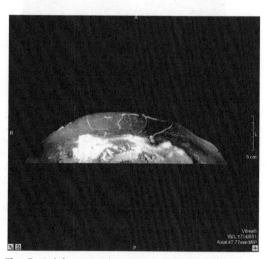

Fig. 3. Axial magnetic resonance image. The arrow shows the left side dominant perforator with its branching to the contralateral side.

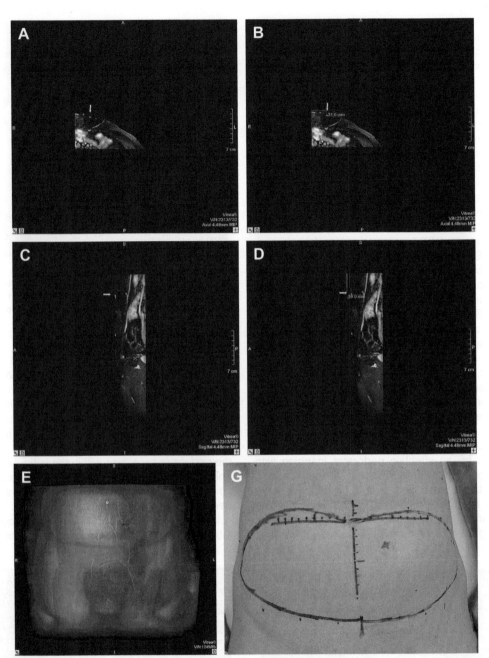

Fig. 4. (*A*) Axial magnetic resonance image showing the chosen perforator. The arrow indicates the point at which the perforator arises from the muscle. (*B*) We measure the distance from the midline to the perforator in the axial view, and this is given the value *x*. (*C*) Sagittal magnetic resonance image showing the chosen perforator. The arrow indicates the point at which the perforator arises from the muscle. (*D*) The second measure is done in the sagittal view measuring from the umbilicus level to the exit of the perforator. This is the *y* value. (*E*) MRI 3D reconstruction for the same patient. The 2 points represent umbilicus level and indicate where the perforator pierces the fascia. (*F*) These values are transferred from the computer to a preoperative form for abdominal flap planning and to the skin, and we locate the exact point where we will find the perforator when we raise the flap. (*G*) Preoperative markings with the dominant perforator located.

F

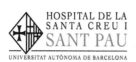

HOSPITAL DE LA
SANTA CREU I
SANT PAU
UNIVERSITAT AUTÒNOMA DE BARCELONA

**Plastic Surgery
Department**

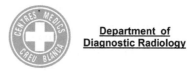

**Department of
Diagnostic Radiology**

MRI FOR PERFORATOR ABDOMINAL FLAPS

Patient details:
Date:

RIGHT DIEPs

DEEP	X	Y	SUPERFICIAL	X	Y	CALIBER	COURSE
1							
2							
3							

LEFT DIEPs

DEEP	X	Y	SUPERFICIAL	X	Y	CALIBER	COURSE
1	3.1	-3.9					
2							
3							

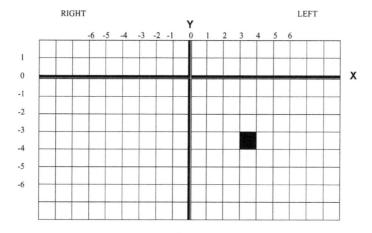

COMMENTS:

- DIEA INTRAMUSCULAR COURSE:

- SIEA/V ASSESSMENT:

- OTHERS:

Fig. 4. (continued)

in definition of the perforator intramuscular course. However, with the MR angiography (MRA) technique FBI, we obtained a better definition of the perforator intramuscular course in all cases, and we were also able to assess the reliability of the superficial inferior epigastric system and its vascular connections with the deep system. As a result, we have since performed the preoperative study of patients having breast reconstruction with non–contrast-enhanced MR angiography technique FBI.[26]

The first step with this technique is to acquire multiplanar images with the patients supine; the same position as they will be placed at surgery. No prior patient preparation is needed. We use high-speed parallel imaging (speeder technology) to achieve accelerated scan times. Initially, sagittal scouts are acquired to locate the inferior abdominal wall and to delimit the study zone. A sequence phase 3D+5_FSfbi is used in the anterior coronal plane with the following parameters: TR, 2694; TE, 80; slice thickness, 1.5 mm; number of slices, 50; number of acquisitions, 1; 512×512 matrix; field of view, 380×380 mm; TI, 160; and resp+ECG gate. A sequence phase 3D+5_FSfbi is then performed in the axial plane with the following parameters: TR, 2900; TE, 78; slice thickness, 3 mm; number of slices, 56; number of acquisitions, 1; 704×704 matrix; field of view, 380×380 mm; TI, 160; and resp+ECG gate. The anterior coronal plane phase only includes the anterior abdominal wall, from a plane immediately below the pubis to the xiphoid process of the sternum. The axial plane phase includes the area from the infrapubic zone to 3 cm above the umbilicus. The acquisition time ranges from 10 to 20 minutes. Multiplanar formatted images and 3D volume rendered images are regenerated on a Vitrea computer workstation (Vitrea version 3.0.1. Vital Images, Plymouth, MN, USA).

The images obtained are interpreted by both the radiologist and the plastic surgeon who is going to harvest the DIEP flap. The team chooses the perforator considered the most suitable according to the following criteria: largest caliber, best location, and shortest intramuscular course. The perforator selected gives a pair of x/y coordinates based on an axial system centered on the umbilicus and the flap can be raised based on the dominant perforator. The surgeon is provided with 3 types of image: axial, sagittal, and coronal.

The axial views and sagittal reconstructions are of great help in the assessment of the perforator vessel to evaluate its dependence on the main trunk or any direct branch of the deep inferior epigastric artery and to delimit its origin on the fascia and its distribution through subcutaneous fat and skin. Rendered reconstructions allow us to mark on the patient's skin the exact point where the perforator vessel emerges through the fascia of the rectus abdominis muscle. When we choose the best the perforator in the imaging technique, we look for the point where it pierces the fascia in the axial view and we mark an arrow on the skin at this level. From there, the arrow will appear in all views. We draw a coordinate x/y axis on the umbilicus and we make measurements to locate the exit of the perforating vessel in relation to the umbilicus. First, we measure the distance from the midline to the perforator in the axial view, and this is given the value x. The second measure is done in the sagittal view, measuring from the umbilicus level to the exit of the perforator. This

is the y value. If we transfer these values from the computer to paper, we locate the exact point where we will find the perforator when we raise the flap. Before we complete the study with the radiologist, we like to look at the coronal cuts to assess the connections between the superficial and deep systems and visualize the subcutaneous and branching pattern of the deep inferior epigastric arterial system (**Fig. 4**).

DISCUSSION

Raising a perforator flap requires meticulous dissection of the perforator vessels, sparing the muscle structure with its segmentary motor nerves. Special skill is needed for such surgical dissection, and the intraoperative time is considerable. Because the vascular anatomy of the abdominal wall varies greatly among individuals and even between one hemiabdomen and another in the same individual, establishing a vascular map of each patient before surgery facilitates dissection.

The ability to detect the dominant perforating artery before surgery saves considerable time for the surgeon. The benefits thus extend to the patient and also to reducing costs and conserving resources. Many techniques have been used to preoperatively map abdominal perforating vessels. The ideal technique should possess low cost, high availability and reproducibility, and high reliability in selecting the dominant perforator. In addition, it should be fast to perform, easy to interpret, and free of morbidity.[27]

The financial cost is complex and has not yet been evaluated. The cost of the imaging alone is variable, but is in the order of US$250 for a duplex ultrasound, US$400 for CTA, and US$600 for MRA in the USA.[10] In Europe, the cost of a MDCT and MRI ranges between 250 and 450 Euros. However, these costs are only significant in the context of cost savings from the reduction in operating time and length of stay, which have all been shown to be reduced with the use of CTA or MRA.

In recent years, the MDCT has been increasingly used in perforator vessel mapping and highly accepted by world-renowned microsurgical teams.[15–22,28–30] The advantage of this technique is that it is reliable and accurate in selecting the best abdominal perforating vessels and, furthermore, it provides images that are easy to interpret. Data obtained using MDCT enable surgeons to select a dissection strategy. The dominant perforator vessel can be chosen before surgery not only by its caliber but also on grounds of its route and anatomic relationships with surrounding structures. This capability makes the procedure safer and faster. As a result, the surgical time required for the flap harvest has decreased significantly, as have postoperative complication rates.[15,31] However, an important drawback is that the patient receives an extra radiation dose, comparable with a routine abdominal CT scan. In addition, the intravenous contrast medium, necessary to obtain high-resolution images, can produce patient discomfort and even severe systemic allergic reactions as well as contrast extravasations.[23,24]

To overcome the limitations of MDCT, we began to search for an MRI technique for preoperative perforators mapping. In 2005, we started out with a 1.5-T MR system because this technology is available in most hospitals and it does not produce any radiation. The main drawbacks compared with MDCT were that the new technique was time consuming, three-dimensional reconstruction was not of good quality, and a precise analysis of the perforators' intramuscular course and its anatomic relationships was not possible. Because of these limitations, after the first short case series, we decided not to continue this kind of 1.5-T MRI in preoperative perforators mapping. Other investigators also found these same drawbacks in their preliminary experience using this technique. They concluded that MRI plays a role in the imaging of abdominal perforators, but that CT scan was still the preferred modality.[24,32]

In 2007, we found that SSFP image acquisition sequencing with the 1.5-T MRI yielded high-resolution images with no need for intravenous contrast. Moreover, in 2008, the new image acquisition sequence, obtained with noncontrast 1.5-T

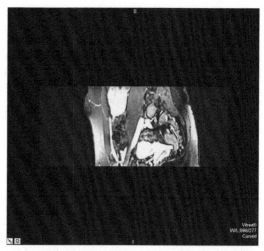

Fig. 5. Sagittal magnetic resonance image. The deep inferior epigastric systems and a dominant perforator with its intramuscular course and its branching to the surface can be seen.

MR angiography using the FBI technique, provided a further notable improvement. With this technique, we can see the perforating vessel's intramuscular course (**Fig. 5**), its anatomic relationships with the surrounding structures, and its branching within the flap in a way that no other technique has allowed so far.

Noncontrast 1.5-T MRI has proved to be highly valuable in abdominal perforator mapping. It accurately assesses the abdominal wall microcirculation, enabling us to choose the appropriate dominant perforator (**Fig. 6**). According to our intraoperative findings, it provides 100% reliability in selecting the most suitable perforator. This

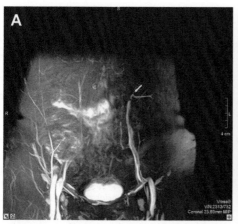
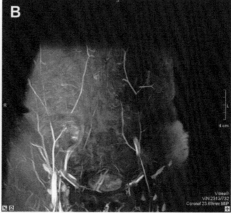

Fig. 6. (A) Coronal magnetic resonance image showing the abdominal vascular network (deep layer). The arrow indicates the dominant perforator arising from the muscle through the subcutaneous tissue. (B) Coronal magnetic resonance image showing the abdominal vascular network (superficial layer). The arrow indicates the course of the dominant perforator through the subcutaneous tissue.

reliability is the same as with MDCT, according to the literature.[15-20,33] Acquisition time ranges from 15 to 20 minutes; although this is longer than the MDCT, we consider it acceptable given that the patient is not radiated. Since we have been using this technique, we have also found a clear decrease in the number of postoperative complications, particularly those concerning partial necrosis of the flap.

SUMMARY

In search of an optimal perforator mapping method, we have found that the 1.5-T noncontrast MRI FBI technique not only provides reliable information on the vascular anatomy of the abdominal wall and identifies the precise localization of the dominant perforator, as with MDCT, but avoids radiation to the patient and eliminates the need for intravenous medium.

This new technique can be considered an ideal method for preoperative planning of breast reconstruction with DIEP flaps. However, despite the usefulness of this technique in daily practice, we continue to use the CT scan in cases of delayed reconstruction, because the perforator vessels can be studied in these circumstances as part of the extension study requested by the oncologist. In most cases, the decision to perform MRI or CT is determined by the availability of the radiology department.

REFERENCES

1. Allen RJ, Treece P. Deep inferior epigastric perforator flap for breast reconstruction. Ann Plast Surg 1994;32:32–8.
2. Craigie JE, Allen RJ. Autogenous breast reconstruction with the deep inferior epigastric perforator flap. Clin Plast Surg 2003;30:359–69.
3. Granzow JW, Levine JL. Breast reconstruction with the deep inferior epigastric perforator flap: history and an update on current technique. J Plast Reconstr Aesthet Surg 2006;59:571–9.
4. Blondeel PN, Boeckx WD. Refinements in free flap breast reconstruction: the free bilateral deep inferior epigastric perforator flap anastomosed to internal mammary artery. Br J Plast Surg 1994;47:495–501.
5. Blondeel PN, Neligan PC. Complications: avoidance and treatment. In: Blondeel PN, Morris SF, Hallock GG, et al, editors. Perforator flaps: anatomy, technique and clinical applications. St Louis (MO): Quality Medical Publishing; 2006. p. 118–9. Chapter 7.
6. Masia J, Larrañaga J, Clavero JA, et al. The value of the multidetector row computed tomography for the preoperative planning of deep inferior epigastric perforator flap: our experience in 162 cases. Ann Plast Surg 2008;60:29–36.
7. Tregaskiss AP, Goodwin AN, Acland RD. The cutaneous arteries of the anterior abdominal wall: a three-dimensional study. Plast Reconstr Surg 2007;120:442–50.
8. Vandevoort M, Vranckx JJ, Fabre G. Perforator topography of the deep inferior epigastric perforator flap in 100 cases of breast reconstruction. Plast Reconstr Surg 2002;109:1912–8.
9. Giunta RE, Geisweid A, Feller MD. The value of preoperative Doppler sonography for planning free perforator flaps. Plast Reconstr Surg 2000;105:2381–6.
10. Rozen WM, Anavekar NS, Ashton MW, et al. Does the preoperative imaging of perforators with CT angiography improve operative outcomes in breast reconstruction? Microsurgery 2008;28(7):516e23.
11. Masia J, Clavero JA, Larrañaga JR, et al. Multidetector-row computed tomography in the planning of abdominal perforator flaps. J Plast Reconstr Aesthet Surg 2006;59:594–9.
12. Blondeel PN, Beyens G, Verhaeghe R, et al. Doppler flowmetry in the planning of perforator flaps. Br J Plast Surg 1998;51:202–9.
13. Taylor GI, Doyle M, McCarten G. The Doppler probe for planning flaps: anatomical study and clinical applications. Br J Plast Surg 1990;43:1–16.
14. Hallock GG. Doppler sonography and color duplex imaging for planning a perforator flap. Clin Plast Surg 2003;30:347–57.
15. Masia J, Clavero JA, Larrañaga J, et al. Preoperative planning of the abdominal perforator flap with multidetector row computed tomography: 3 years of experience. Plast Reconstr Surg 2008;122:80e–1e.
16. Clavero JA, Masia J, Larrañaga J, et al. MDCT in the preoperative planning of abdominal perforator surgery for postmastectomy breast reconstruction. AJR Am J Roentgenol 2008;191:670–6.
17. Masia J, Clavero JA, Carrera A. Planificación preoperatoria de los colgajos de perforantes. Cir Plas Iberolatinoam 2006;32:237–42.
18. Masia J, Clavero JA. Multidetector row CT in the planning of abdominal perforator flaps. In: Blondeel PN, Morris SF, Hallock GG, et al, editors. Perforator flaps: anatomy, techniques and clinical applications. St Louis (MO): Quality Medical Publications; 2006. p. 91–114.
19. Masia J, Kosutic D, Clavero JA, et al. Preoperative computed tomographic angiogram for deep inferior epigastric artery perforator flap breast reconstruction. J Reconstr Microsurg 2010;26(1):21–8.
20. Hamdi M, Van Landuyt K, Hedent EV, et al. Advances in autogenous breast reconstruction. The role of preoperative perforator mapping. Ann Plast Surg 2007;58:18–26.

21. Rozen WM, Phillips TJ, Ashton MW, et al. Preoperative imaging for DIEA perforator flaps: a comparative study of computed tomographic angiography and Doppler ultrasound. Plast Reconstr Surg 2008;121:1–8.

22. Martin CJ. Radiation dosimetry for diagnostic medical exposures. Radiat Prot Dosimetry 2008;128:389–412.

23. Cochran ST. Anaphylactoid reactions to radiocontrast media. Curr Allergy Asthma Rep 2005;5:28–31.

24. Cochran ST, Bomyea K, Sayre JW. Trends in adverse events after I.V. administration of contrast media. AJR Am J Roentgenol 2001;176:1385–8.

25. Alonso-Burgos A, García-Tutor E, Bastarrika G, et al. Preoperative planning of DIEP and SGAP flaps: preliminary experience with magnetic resonance angiography using 3-Tesla equipment and blood-pool contrast medium. J Plast Reconstr Aesthet Surg 2010;63(2):298–304.

26. Masia J, Kosuotic D, Cervelli D, et al. In search of the ideal method in perforator mapping: noncontrast magnetic resonance imaging. J Reconstr Microsurg 2010;26(1):29–35.

27. Smit JM, Klein S, Werker PM. An overview of methods for vascular mapping in the planning of free flaps. J Plast Reconstr Aesthet Surg 2010;63(9):e674–82.

28. Mun GH, Kim HJ, Cha MK, et al. Impact of perforator mapping using multidetector-row computed tomographic angiography on free thoracodorsal artery perforator flap transfer. Plast Reconstr Surg 2008;122:1079–88.

29. Imai R, Matsumura H, Tanaka K, et al. Comparison of Doppler sonography and multidetector-row computed tomography in the imaging findings of the deep inferior epigastric perforator artery. Ann Plast Surg 2008;61:94–8.

30. Pacifico MD, See MS, Cavale M, et al. Preoperative planning for DIEP breast reconstruction: early experience of the use of computerised tomography angiography with VoNavix 3D software for perforator navigation. J Plast Reconstr Aesthet Surg 2009; 62(11):1464–9.

31. Smit JM, Dimopoulou A, Liss AG, et al. Preoperative CT angiography reduces surgery time in perforator flap reconstruction. J Plast Reconstr Aesthet Surg 2009;62:1112–7.

32. Rozen WM, Stella DL, Bowden J, et al. Advances in the pre-operative planning of deep inferior epigastric artery perforator flaps: magnetic resonance angiography. Microsurgery 2009;29:119–23.

33. Neil-Dwyer JG, Ludman CN, Schaverien M, et al. Magnetic resonance angiography in preoperative planning of deep inferior epigastric artery perforator flaps. J Plast Reconstr Aesthet Surg 2009;62(12):1661–5.

Contrast-Enhanced Magnetic Resonance Angiography

Julie V. Vasile, MD[a,b,c,]*, Tiffany M. Newman, MD[d],
Martin R. Prince, MD, PhD[d], David G. Rusch, MD[d,e],
David T. Greenspun, MD[a,c], Robert J. Allen, MD[a,c],
Joshua L. Levine, MD[a,c]

KEYWORDS

- Autologous perforator flap breast reconstruction
- Magnetic resonance angiography • Imaging • DIEP flap
- SIEA flap • Gluteal artery perforator • TUG flap

Preoperative anatomic imaging of vasculature markedly enhances the ability of a surgeon to devise a surgical strategy before going to the operating room. Before the era of preoperative perforator imaging, a surgeon had little knowledge of an individual patient's vascular anatomy until surgery was well under way. As a result, perforator selection could be a tedious decision process that occurred in the operating room at the expense of operating time and general anesthetic requirement.

The authors' favored modality for preoperative imaging has changed as technology has advanced. Initially only a hand-held Doppler ultrasound was used. A Doppler ultrasound is portable and simple to use, but cannot differentiate perforating vessels from superficial and deep axial vessels or robust perforators from miniscule ones, accurately locate perforators that do not exit perpendicular from the fascia, or provide information on the anatomic course of a vessel.[1,2] By comparison, color Duplex sonography provides more detailed information about the anatomy of the vessels, but requires highly trained technicians with knowledge of perforator anatomy and is time consuming.[2] The technique's most crucial drawback is an inability to produce anatomic images in a format that a surgeon can easily and independently view. As a result, the authors do not use this modality for imaging perforator flaps in their patients.

Computed tomographic angiography (CTA) is a modality that can demonstrate vessel anatomy, assess vessel caliber, accurately locate perforators, and produce anatomic images in a format that a surgeon can easily and independently view. Although CTA can be performed quickly in as little as 15 minutes,[1,2] patients must be exposed to ionizing radiation. Recent articles in the medical literature and lay press warn that physicians may be exposing patients to excessive and potentially unnecessary radiation, and question the long-term effects of such exposure.[3,4] Patients with breast cancer often have a heightened concern for any factor that can potentially increase the risk of developing a second cancer and may perceive the risks of radiation exposure

Disclosure: Dr Prince has patent agreements with GE, Siemens, Phillips, Hitachi, Toshiba, Bracco, Bayer, Epix, Lantheus, Mallinckrodt, Medrad, Nemoto, and Topspins.
[a] Department of Plastic Surgery, New York Eye and Ear Infirmary, 310 East 14th Street, New York, NY 10003, USA
[b] Department of Surgery, Stamford Hospital, 30 Shelburne Road, Stamford, CT 06902, USA
[c] Center for Microsurgical Breast Reconstruction, 1776 Broadway, Suite 1200, New York, NY 10019, USA
[d] Department of Radiology, Weil Cornell Imaging at New York Presbyterian Hospital, Weil Cornell and Columbia University, 416 East 55th Street, New York, NY 10022, USA
[e] Department of Radiology, White Plains Hospital, 41 East Post Road, White Plains, NY 10461, USA
* Corresponding author. 1290 Summer Street, Suite 3200, Stamford, CT 06905.
E-mail address: jvasilemd@gmail.com

Clin Plastic Surg 38 (2011) 263–275
doi:10.1016/j.cps.2011.03.008

even more negatively. A subset of patients with breast cancer gene (BRCA) mutations, which confer an increased risk of developing both breast and ovarian cancer, are especially concerned about receiving radiation to the abdomen. Furthermore, iodinated contrast for CTA has been associated with small, but real risks of anaphylaxis and nephrotoxicity.[5,6]

The dose of radiation from one chest radiograph (0.1 millisieverts [mSv]) is relatively low and is approximately equivalent to the dose of environmental radiation one receives by virtue of living on earth for 10 days.[7] By comparison, a computed tomography (CT) scan of the abdomen delivers 6 to 10 mSv of radiation, which is approximately equivalent to 3 years of environmental radiation.[1,3,7] Controversy lies in the amount of radiation needed for cancer induction, but experts agree that unnecessary exposure to ionizing radiation should be avoided. Frequently the diagnostic utility of CT outweighs the uncertain, low risk of cancer induction.[8] However, the authors believe that alternative methods of vascular imaging should be employed whenever possible, and this led them to consider MRA (magnetic resonance angiography) as an imaging modality.

Magnetic resonance imaging (MRI) works by using a magnetic field to uniformly align the spin of hydrogen atoms in tissue. The subsequent application of a radiofrequency pulse results in release of energy as hydrogen atoms return to their relaxed state. MRI coils detect the released energy, and computer software processes the data into anatomic images. Exposure to a magnetic field or radiofrequency pulse with MRI has not been linked to the development of cancer.[9] A paramagnetic contrast agent (gadolinium-containing) is injected to enhance vessels. Because MRI does not use radiation, multiple series of images can be obtained. Vessels usually are first imaged in the arterial phase, and subsequently the arterial/venous phase for visualization of the artery and vein together. Additional series of images are acquired to view the vasculature in multiple planes: axial, coronal, and sagittal.

Gadolinium-containing contrast agents used for MRA have several distinct advantages over iodinated contrast agents used for CTA. The incidence of an acute allergic reaction to iodinated contrast is 3%, which is orders of magnitude higher than the 0.07% incidence of allergic reaction to gadolinium contrast.[5,10] Furthermore, unlike gadolinium contrast agents, iodinated CT contrast agents can induce renal insufficiency even in patients with normal renal function.[6,11]

Gadolinium contrast agents can potentially induce nephrogenic systemic fibrosis (NSF), also called nephrogenic fibrosing dermopathy.

However, reports of NSF have been limited to patients with impaired renal function.[12–14] Patients with an acute kidney injury or chronic severe renal disease (glomerular filtration rate <30 mL/min/1.73 m^2) are considered most at risk.[12] NSF is a very rare disease, with about 330 cases reported worldwide.[13,14] Although patients undergoing elective microsurgical free flap are generally healthy and thus are not at significant risk for developing NSF, a creatinine level is drawn preoperatively in patients with a history of hypertension, diabetes, renal disease, or any other indication that renal function may be impaired.

Disadvantages of MRA are contraindication to use with a cardiac pacemaker or in very claustrophobic patients. However, none of the authors' patients have been excluded from MRA imaging because of these factors. Continuing advances in MRA have decreased the procedure time for a single donor site to as little as 20 minutes and have decreased the actual acquisition scan time to 20 seconds.[15,16]

MRA is currently the favored modality for preoperative imaging because the authors have found the accuracy to be on par with CTA. With their first MRA protocol developed in 2006, in 50 abdominal flaps, the authors found that the location of the perforating vessel correlated with the intraoperative findings within 1 cm in 100% of the flaps, the relative size (ie, comparing size of one vessel to another for the same patient) of the perforators visualized on MRA correlated with the intraoperative findings in 100% of the flaps, all relatively large perforators visualized on MRA were found at surgery (0% false positive), and intraoperative perforators of significant size were visualized on MRA in 96% of the flaps (4% false negative).[17] By comparison, a study using preoperative CTA on 36 patients found 0% false-positive and 0% false-negative results.[1] Another study using preoperative CTA in 42 patients found one false-positive and one false-negative result.[18] The 2 false-negative results in the authors' original study were due to inadequate visualization of lateral row perforators secondary to signal interference from the thigh and buttock fat.

METHODS

Refinements in the authors' MRA protocol were made in 2008.[17,19,20] The switch was made to a 1.5-T scanner to eliminate inhomogeneous fat suppression associated with a 3-T magnet, for improved visualization of lateral row perforators. In addition, gadobenate dimeglumine (Bracco, Princeton, NJ, USA), a gadolinium-based contrast agent that binds to albumin and has a longer half-life in the bloodstream, was used to extend the craniocaudal field of view. Furthermore, the authors took advantage of the lack of radiation exposure to do serial image acquisitions with a patient in the prone and then supine position. The result of these modifications is that abdominal, gluteal, and upper thigh perforators can be visualized in one study. Also, 3-dimensional (3D) reconstruction was used to view the vessels on surface-rendered images for improved understanding of perforator location.

First, patients were scanned in the prone position because the quality of the images of the abdominal wall perforators is superior to those obtained in the supine position. Respiratory motion is reduced in the prone position and motion artifact is minimized, which enhances abdominal perforator assessment. Fascia is a stable structure in the abdomen, and the location of the abdominal perforators in reference to the base of the umbilical stalk is not affected by the prone position. By contrast, the curved anatomy of the buttock is greatly distorted in the supine position, and buttock perforator location in reference to the gluteal crease is significantly affected. Finally, patients were scanned in the supine position to estimate abdominal flap volume and reconfirm abdominal perforator location.

MRA images and the associated radiology report were reviewed by the surgeon and an optimal perforator(s) was selected. Intraoperative vessel assessment was compared with vessel assessment on MRA, as described in previous articles.[17,19] Immediately after surgery, surveys were completed by the operating surgeon.

PATIENTS

Thirty-seven consecutive patients were imaged with MRA from August 2008 to June 2009. The inclusion criterion was that all patients referred for breast reconstruction were able to travel to the one radiological center that used the authors' MRA protocol. Patients located in other states who could not travel were excluded. Exclusion criterion was inability to undergo MRA examination (cardiac pacemaker, severe claustrophobia, and severe renal insufficiency), for which no patients were excluded.

RESULTS

Sixty-two abdominal, gluteal, thigh, and lumbar flaps were used for breast reconstruction in 37 patients. **Table 1** illustrates the type of flap and type of perforator used.

The new MRA protocol improved the quality of the images and accuracy of perforator assessment. The relative vessel size (ie, comparing size of one vessel to another for the same patient) on MRA compared with that found at surgery was accurate in all flaps (100%), the predicted perforator location was accurate to within 0.5 cm in all flaps (100%), and there were no false-positive (all relatively large perforators visualized on MRA were found at surgery) and no false-negative results (intraoperative perforators of significant size were all visualized on MRA).

The preoperatively selected vessel was used in all patients except in 2 cases. In the first case, a backup inferior gluteal artery perforator (IGAP) vessel was used instead of a planned deep femoral artery perforator (DFAP) in an inferior buttock flap. The IGAP vessel was identified first intraoperatively by the surgeon, and was of adequate caliber, and thus dissected. In the second case, a second small deep inferior epigastric perforator (DIEP) was added to a preoperatively selected large DIEP because it lined up without necessitating an

Table 1
Type of flap and type of perforator(s) used

Flap Type	Number of Flaps	Single Intramuscular Perforator	Double Intramuscular Perforator	Septocutaneous Vessel
DIEP	48	37	9[a]	2
SIEA	1			
SGAP	5	3		2
LAP	1			1
IGAP	2	2[a]		
DFAP	4			4
TUG without muscle	1			1

Abbreviations: DFAP, deep femoral artery perforator; DIEP, deep inferior epigastric perforator; IGAP, inferior gluteal artery perforator; LAP, lumbar artery perforator; SGAP, superior gluteal artery perforator; SIEA, superficial inferior epigastric artery; TUG, transverse upper gracilis.

[a] All preoperatively selected vessels were used to carry the flap, except in one patient a second small DIEP was added to a large preoperatively selected DIEP, and in a second patient a backup IGAP was used instead of a DFAP.

incision through rectus muscle fibers. The second small DIEP was in retrospect visualized on MRA, but not included in the MRA radiology report because the diameter was less than 1 mm.

The design of abdominal flaps was moved cephalad or caudal to capture the best perforator in 20 of 29 patients (69%). In 20 abdominal flaps, the flap weight estimated from MRA differed from the actual flap weight at surgery by an average of 47 g. MRA determined the design of all buttock flaps (100%). MRA determined the selection of which thigh (ipsilateral or contralateral) was used for a unilateral breast reconstruction.

DISCUSSION ON THE FINER POINTS OF MRA AND PERFORATOR SELECTION

Vessel caliber in conjunction with a centralized location on the flap is the most important factor for optimal perforator selection at every donor site. Caliber measurements are uniformly performed at the point where a vessel exits the

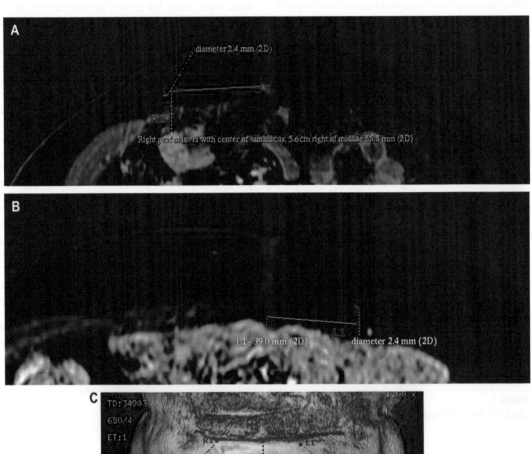

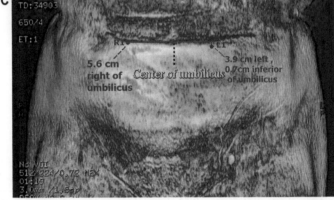

Fig. 1. (A) Axial MRA of perforator R1. Location is measured in reference to the base of the center of the umbilical stalk. (B) Axial MRA of perforator L1. Diameter is measured at the point where the perforator exits the anterior rectus fascia. (C) Surface-rendered 3-dimensional (3D) reconstruction MRA. Location of perforators is in reference to the umbilicus.

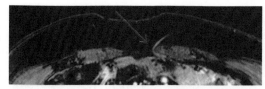

Fig. 2. Axial MRA. Arrow points to septocutaneous perforator. (*From* Greenspun D, Vasile J, Levine JL, et al. Anatomic imaging of abdominal perforator flaps without ionizing radiation: seeing is believing with magnetic resonance imaging angiography. J Reconstr Microsurg 2010;26(1):41; with permission.)

superficial fascia. Location measurements are performed in reference to a landmark at each donor site. Specific considerations regarding each donor site are presented here.

Abdomen

The location of the vessel on exiting the anterior rectus fascia is measured in reference to the center of the base of the umbilical stalk for improved accuracy, as seen in **Fig. 1**. Vessel caliber measurements are also performed just

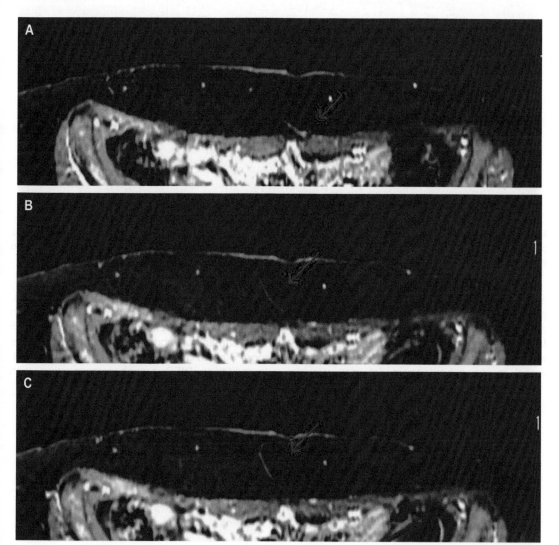

Fig. 3. (*A*) Axial MRA. Arrow points to medial row perforator. (*B*) Axial MRA. Arrow points to arborization of the same perforator crossing the midline. (*C*) Axial MRA. Arrow points to further arborization of the same perforator.

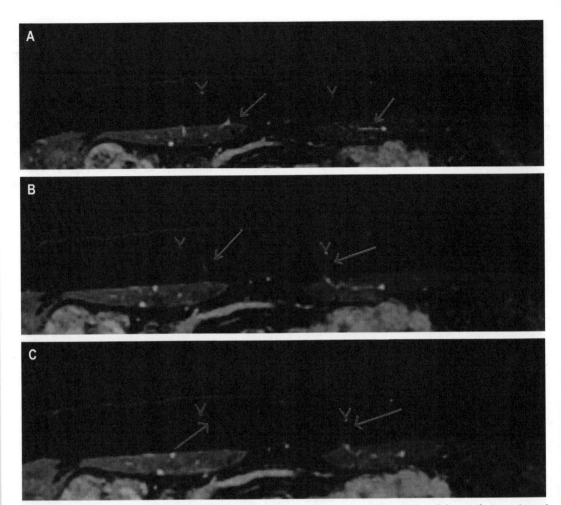

Fig. 4. "V" denotes superficial inferior epigastric vein (SIEV), and arrows point to bilateral deep inferior epigastric perforators (DIEPs). (*A*) Axial MRA. (*B*) Axial MRA. Left DIEP meeting SIEV. (*C*) Axial MRA. Right DIEP branch also meeting SIEV.

above the anterior rectus fascia level. An intramuscular course length or a septocutaneous course, as seen in **Fig. 2**, can add important information for a surgeon to anticipate a tedious or straightforward dissection. Also, the branching pattern of the vessel in the subcutaneous fat may provide valuable information. In a unilateral reconstruction, it is helpful to see a medial row perforator with branches crossing into the subcutaneous fat on the contralateral abdomen, because zone III is more likely to be well perfused, as seen in **Fig. 3**. In addition, DIEP branches connecting with

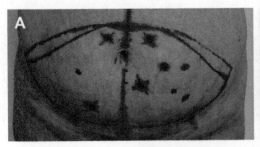
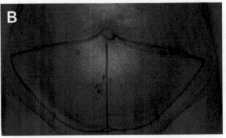

Fig. 5. (*A*) Abdominal flap design shifted cephalad to capture the 2 largest perforators located above the umbilicus. (*B*) Abdominal flap design shifted caudal.

superficial inferior epigastric venous branches may theoretically provide improved venous drainage. An example of a DIEP connecting with a superficial inferior epigastric vein branch is seen in **Fig. 4**.[21]

The detailed information on vasculature provided by MRA influences flap design. As a result of imaging, the design of abdominal flaps was moved cephalad or caudal to capture the best perforator in 20 of 29 patients (69%). Pictures of two different flap designs are seen in **Fig. 5**.

Helpful images that a radiologist can add to the study are coronal images, which best show the branching pattern of the deep inferior epigastric system, as seen in **Fig. 6**. Also, 3D reconstructed images are useful in examining for a common origin of the superficial inferior epigastric artery with the superficial circumflex iliac artery, as seen in **Fig. 7**. However, a superficial inferior epigastric artery was rarely used because a DIEP with adequate caliber and location was usually found. In the authors' study, 48 DIEP (98%) and 1 superficial inferior epigastric artery (SIEA) (2%) vessels were used. In the one case that a SIEA was used, a contralateral SIEA was added to augment perfusion in a unilateral DIEP flap breast reconstruction, in which zone III and a portion of zone IV of the abdomen required additional perfusion.

Volume-rendered 3D reconstructions can be performed by a radiologist to add important information on the projected abdominal flap weight, as seen in **Fig. 8**. First, a radiologist has to be trained in the typical markings and dimensions of an abdominal flap to increase accuracy. In 20 abdominal flaps, the flap weight estimated from MRA differed from the actual flap weight at surgery by an average of 47 g.[20,22] The weight difference can be attributed to several causes: the mean density of fat (0.92) was used in the volume calculation, but the abdominal flap also contains skin and vessels; the actual flap dimensions marked by a surgeon will differ from those made by

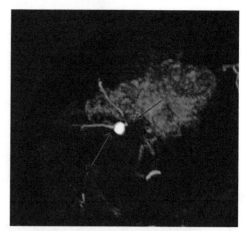

Fig. 7. 3D Reconstruction MRA. Arrows point to separate origin of the superficial inferior epigastric artery and superficial circumflex iliac artery. (*From* Greenspun D, Vasile J, Levine JL, et al. Anatomic imaging of abdominal perforator flaps without ionizing radiation: seeing is believing with magnetic resonance imaging angiography. J Reconstr Microsurg 2010; 26(1):43; with permission.)

a radiologist; beveling of extra subcutaneous fat outside the marked dimension during surgery was sometimes performed; and extra tissue was taken outside the marked dimension to harvest an inguinal lymph node with 2 DIEP flaps for lymph node transfer in 2 patients with mastectomy and upper extremity lymphedema.

Buttock

A photograph of the marked top of the gluteal crease is included in the radiology report for increased accuracy, as seen in **Fig. 9**. The location of the vessel on exiting the superficial fascia is measured in reference to the top of the gluteal crease along the curved skin contour of the buttock with the patient in the prone position for increased accuracy, as seen in **Fig. 10**. Surface-rendered 3D reconstruction is invaluable to the surgeon for location of perforators because of the curved contour of the buttock.

The placement of the buttock flap skin paddle is also significantly influenced by optimal perforator

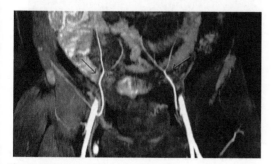

Fig. 6. Coronal MRA. The branching pattern of the deep inferior epigastric system is visualized. Arrows point to bifurcation of deep inferior epigastric vessels bilaterally.

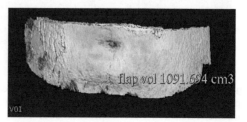

Fig. 8. Volume-rendered 3D reconstruction MRA. Abdominal flap volume measured by the radiologist.

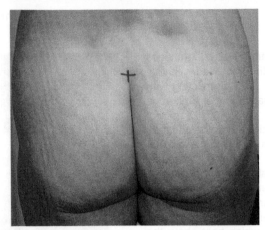

Fig. 9. Top of gluteal crease is the reference point marked by the radiologist.

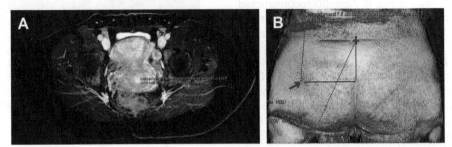

Fig. 10. (*A*) Axial MRA. Gluteal perforator location is measured along the curved skin surface. (*B*) Surface-rendered 3D reconstruction MRA. Same perforator located on the buttock, in reference to top of gluteal crease. (*From* Vasile JV, Newman T, Rusch DG, et al. Anatomic imaging of gluteal perforator flaps without ionizing radiation: seeing is believing with magnetic resonance angiography. J Reconstr Microsurg 2010;26(1):48; with permission.)

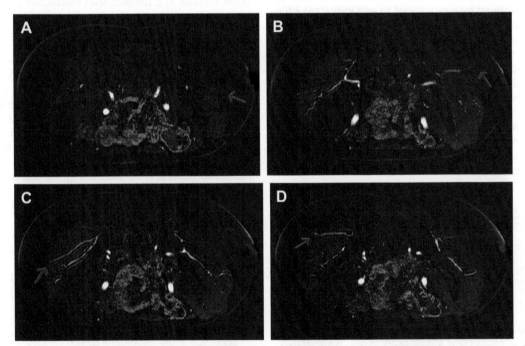

Fig. 11. Arrows point to laterally and cephalad located perforators on the same patient. (*A*) Axial MRA. Right septocutaneous superior gluteal artery perforator (SGAP). (*B*) Axial MRA. Right intramuscular double branching SGAP. (*C*) Axial MRA. Left septocutaneous SGAP. (*D*) Axial MRA. Left intramuscular SGAP. (*From* Vasile JV, Newman T, Rusch DG, et al. Anatomic imaging of gluteal perforator flaps without ionizing radiation: seeing is believing with magnetic resonance angiography. J Reconstr Microsurg 2010;26(1):53; with permission.)

location. The goal is to design a flap that incorporates the optimal perforator and a back up option. Because there are usually many large-caliber perforator options in the buttock, vessel location is an important determining factor in selecting the optimal vessel. Laterally positioned perforators will result in more lateral flaps that may spare the central aesthetic unit in superior buttock flaps or the medial cushioning fat in lower buttock flaps. In bilateral flaps, an attempt is made to design flaps that will result in symmetric scars. Examples are shown in **Figs. 11 to 14**.

A benefit of precise knowledge of a patient's vascular anatomy is the ability and confidence to design flaps based on vessels not previously used. **Figs. 13** and **14** illustrate an MRA of a DFAP, which can be advantageous because it usually results in a more laterally and caudally positioned lower buttock flap. In addition, DFAPs are usually septocutaneous after piercing the adductor magnus muscle proximally.[19] In addition, **Fig. 15** illustrates the MRA and flap design of a lumbar artery perforator (LAP) flap, which can be positioned more superiorly to better spare the central aesthetic unit in the buttock and is usually septocutaneous.

Thigh

The design of a medial upper thigh (transverse upper gracilis; TUG) flap is usually fairly standard, and designed to incorporate branches coursing

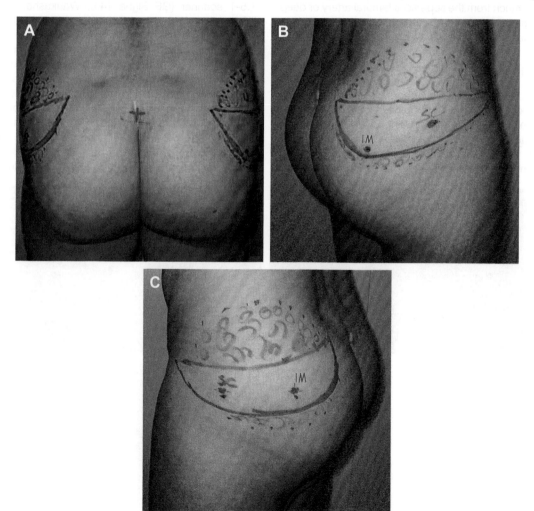

Fig. 12. Flaps designed to incorporate the septocutaneous and backup intramuscular SGAP shown in **Fig. 11.** Septocutaneous perforator is marked "SC" and intramuscular perforator is marked "IM." Planned harvest of subcutaneous fat outside the flap design is marked. (*A*) Posterior buttock. Note that flaps are positioned laterally to spare central aesthetic unit. (*B*) Right oblique buttock. (*C*) Left oblique buttock. (*From* Vasile JV, Newman T, Rusch DG, et al. Anatomic imaging of gluteal perforator flaps without ionizing radiation: seeing is believing with magnetic resonance angiography. J Reconstr Microsurg 2010;26(1):54; with permission.)

through the gracilis muscle from the medial circumflex femoral artery, located 10 cm caudal to the pubic tubercle. Usually a portion of the gracilis muscle is harvested in a TUG flap. However, upper thigh imaging can yield very useful information that can influence surgical planning. **Fig. 16** illustrates an MRA of a septocutaneous perforator from the medial circumflex femoral artery in a patient undergoing a unilateral breast reconstruction. Harvest of this septocutaneous vessel resulted in complete sparing of the gracilis muscle and determined the donor site (ie, which thigh to use for reconstruction). Sometimes a perforator from the medial circumflex femoral artery is large and can be dissected between the gracilis muscle fibers to spare harvesting the gracilis muscle. Moreover, a branch from the superficial femoral artery or deep femoral artery can be used to harvest the same upper thigh tissue and also spare the gracilis muscle.

CURRENT MRA PROTOCOL

In January 2010, the authors switched to a blood pool contrast agent, gadofosveset trisodium (Lantheus Medical Imaging, North Billerica, MA, USA). Gadofosveset trisodium (Ablavar) reversibly binds to albumin with a higher (approximately 90%) binding fraction and effectively stays intravascular

for almost an hour (redistribution half-life = 48 minutes) to allow for excellent-quality images over an expanded examination window.[23,24] Increased imaging quality of the visualization of perforators was immediately noticed, especially through muscle, which can be helpful in determining the intramuscular course.

At the same time the authors switched contrast agents, they came to the realization that the combined arterial venous phase is more useful in selecting the optimal perforator because a perforating artery is paired with a vein, and together they are more easily identified when there is simultaneous enhancement of both vessels.

The most current MRA protocol is as follows. MRA is performed on a long-bore, self-shielded 1.5-T scanner (GE Signa 14.0, Waukasha, WI, USA) using an 8-channel phased-array coil. The field of view extends from 3 cm above the umbilicus to the upper thigh and transversely is set to match the width of the patient. Slice thickness is 3 mm with 1.5-mm overlap. Frequency and reduced field of view shim are adjusted to ensure effective fat suppression over the anterior abdominal fat on precontrast imaging. The first acquisition is started 3 seconds after observation of contrast in the suprarenal aorta (SmartPrep). k-Space is mapped sequentially so the absolute

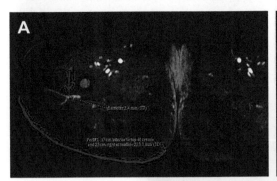
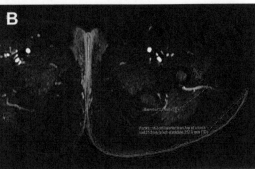
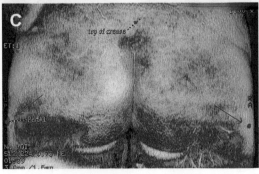

Fig. 13. Arrows point to laterally and caudally located perforators on the same patient. (*A*) Axial MRA. Right septocutaneous deep femoral artery perforator (DFAP). (*B*) Axial MRA. Left septocutaneous DFAP. (*C*) Surface-rendered 3D reconstruction MRA. DFAPs located on buttock skin surface. (*From* Vasile JV, Newman T, Rusch DG, et al. Anatomic imaging of gluteal perforator flaps without ionizing radiation: seeing is believing with magnetic resonance angiography. J Reconstr Microsurg 2010;26(1):49, 50; with permission.)

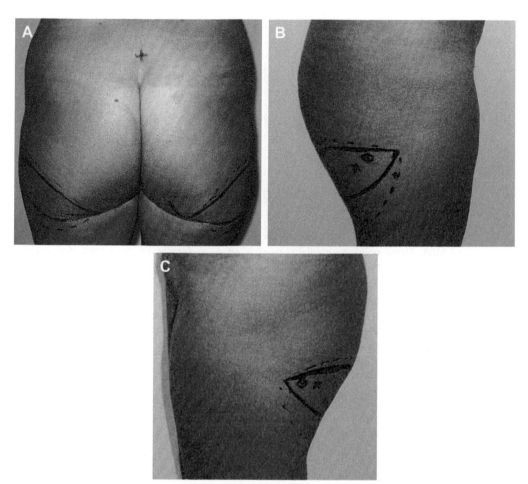

Fig. 14. Flaps designed to incorporate the DFAPs shown in **Fig. 13**. Planned harvest of subcutaneous fat outside the flap is marked with dotted line. (*A*) Posterior buttock. Note that flaps are positioned lateral to spare cushion fat medially. (*B*) Right lateral buttock. (*C*) Left lateral buttock. (*From* Vasile JV, Newman T, Rusch DG, et al. Anatomic imaging of gluteal perforator flaps without ionizing radiation: seeing is believing with magnetic resonance angiography. J Reconstr Microsurg 2010;26(1):51; with permission.)

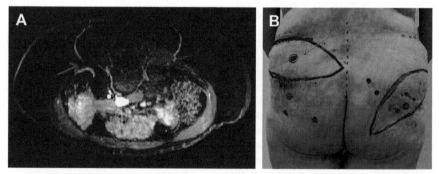

Fig. 15. (*A*) Axial MRA. Arrow points to left lumbar artery perforator (LAP). (*B*) Posterior buttock. Left buttock flap is designed to incorporate LAP (*arrow*). Back up GAP flap was designed, but not used on right buttock. (*From* Vasile JV, Newman T, Rusch DG, et al. Anatomic imaging of gluteal perforator flaps without ionizing radiation: seeing is believing with magnetic resonance angiography. J Reconstr Microsurg 2010;26(1):55; with permission.)

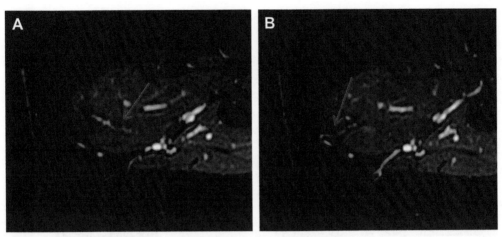

Fig. 16. (*A*) Axial MRA. Arrow points to medial circumflex artery perforator. (*B*) Axial MRA. Arrow points to septocutaneous course of perforator around gracilis muscle.

center of k-space is collected in the middle of the scan (20 seconds after contrast detection). Length of breath-hold is 30 to 35 seconds per acquisition. Repetition time/echo time/flip = 4/1.9/15°. Matrix = 512 × 192–256. Bandwidth = 125 kHz. The injection consists of 10 mL of gadofosveset trisodium at 1 mL/s followed by 20 mL of normal saline. The patient is placed in the prone position for the following sequences: axial and coronal T2-weighted single-shot fast spin echo (SSFSE) images, axial high-resolution 3D liver accelerated volume acquisition (LAVA) pre/during/postdynamic injection of contrast, and postcontrast coronal and sagittal LAVA. The patient is positioned supine for axial high-resolution LAVA. Images are postprocessed on an Advantage Workstation.

This current MRA protocol allows multiple studies in one, and imaging time averages 40 minutes. A patient who unexpectedly is not a candidate for an abdominal perforator flap based on imaging findings, or suddenly changes her preference of donor site, or has a flap failure and requires another perforator flap reconstruction, does not require further studies.

SUMMARY

The tremendous anatomic variability in the vascular system can make perforator flap breast reconstruction challenging for surgeons at all experience levels. Accurate preoperative anatomic vascular imaging enables optimal perforator selection and improves flap design. Shifting the brunt of the perforator selection process preoperatively improves operating efficiency, which can result in reduced operating time, reduced general anesthesia requirements, and potentially increased flap success.[17,25] The authors consider MRA to be the

preoperative method of choice, due to the absence of radiation exposure or iodinated contrast agents and the ability for serial imaging acquisitions to visualize multiple donor site vasculature in one study.

REFERENCES

1. Masia J, Clavero JA, Larranaga JR, et al. Multidetector-row computed tomography in the planning of abdominal perforator flaps. J Plast Reconstr Aesthet Surg 2006;59(6):594–9.
2. Rozen WM, Phillips TJ, Ashton MW, et al. Preoperative imaging for DIEA perforator flaps: a comparative study of computed tomographic angiography and Doppler ultrasound. Plast Reconstr Surg 2008; 121(1):9–16.
3. Brenner DJ, Hall EJ. Computed tomography-an increasing source of radiation exposure. N Engl J Med 2007;357(22):2277–84.
4. Stein R. Too much of a good thing? The growing use of CT scans fuel medical concerns regarding radiation exposure. The Washington Post Newspaper. January 15, 2008.
5. Katayama H, Yamaguchi K, Kozuka T, et al. Adverse reactions to ionic and nonionic contrast media. A report from the Japanese committee on the safety of contrast media. Radiology 1990;175(3):621–8.
6. Parfray P. The clinical epidemiology of contrast-induced nephropathy. Cardiovasc Intervent Radiol 2005;28(Suppl 2):S3–11.
7. Safety in Medical Imaging. American College Radiology Radiological Society North America, Inc. Available at: www.radiologyinfo.org/en/safety/index. cfm?pg=sfty_xray&bhcp=1. Accessed September 27, 2010.
8. Varnholt H. Computed tomography and radiation exposure. N Engl J Med 2008;358(8):852–3.

9. Shellock FG, Crues JV. MR procedures: biologic effects, safety, and patient care. Radiology 2004; 232:635–52.

10. Dillman JR, Ellis JH, Cohan RH, et al. Frequency and severity of acute allergic-like reactions to gadolinium-containing IV contrast media in children and adults. AJR Am J Roentgenol 2007;189:1533–8.

11. Niendorf HP, Alhassan A, Geens VR, et al. Safety review of gadopentetate dimeglumine extended clinical experience after more than five million applications. Invest Radiol 1994;29(Suppl 2):S179–82.

12. FDA drug safety communication: new warnings for using gadolinium-based contrast agents in patients with kidney dysfunction. Available at: http://www.fda.gov/drugs/drugsafety/ucm223966.htm. Accessed September 21, 2010.

13. Cowper SE. Nephrogenic fibrosing dermopathy [ICNSFR Website]. 2001-2009. Available at: http://www.icnsfr.org. Accessed September 22, 2010.

14. Scheinfeld NS, Cowper SE. Nephrogenic fibrosing dermopathy. 2008. Available at: http://www.emedicine.com/derm/topic934.htm. Accessed August 7, 2008.

15. Neil-Dwyer JG, Ludman CN, Schaverien M, et al. Magnetic resonance angiography in preoperative planning of deep inferior epigastric artery perforator flaps. J Plast Reconstr Aesthet Surg 2009; 62:1661–5.

16. Masia J, Kosutic D, Cervelli D, et al. In search of the ideal method in perforator mapping: noncontrast magnetic resonance imaging. J Reconstr Microsurg 2010;26(1):29–35.

17. Greenspun D, Vasile J, Levine JL, et al. Anatomic imaging of abdominal perforator flaps without ionizing radiation: seeing is believing with magnetic resonance imaging angiography. J Reconstr Microsurg 2010;26(1):37–44.

18. Rozen WM, Ashton MW, Stella DL, et al. The accuracy of computed tomographic angiography for mapping the perforators of the deep inferior epigastric artery: a blinded, prospective cohort study. Plast Reconstr Surg 2008;122(4):1003–9.

19. Vasile JV, Newman T, Rusch DG, et al. Anatomic imaging of gluteal perforator flaps without ionizing radiation: seeing is believing with magnetic resonance angiography. J Reconstr Microsurg 2010; 26(1):45–57.

20. Newman TM, Vasile J, Levine JL, et al. Perforator flap magnetic resonance angiography for reconstructive breast surgery: a review of 25 deep inferior epigastric and gluteal perforator artery flap patients. J Magn Reson Imaging 2010;31(5):1176–84.

21. Schaverien MV, Ludman CN, Neil-Dwyer J, et al. Relationship between venous congestion and intra-flap venous anatomy in DIEP flaps using contrast-enhanced magnetic resonance angiography. Plast Reconstr Surg 2010;126(2):385–92.

22. Vasile J, Newman T, Greenspun D. Anatomic vascular imaging of perforator flaps for breast reconstruction: seeing is believing with MRA. Plast Reconstr Surg 2009;124(4S):71.

23. Ersoy H, Jacobs P, Kent CK, et al. Blood pool MR angiography of aortic stent-graft endoleak. AJR Am J Roentgenol 2004;182:1181–6.

24. Klessen C, Hein PA, Huppertz A, et al. First-pass whole-body magnetic resonance angiography (MRA) using the blood-pool contrast medium gadofosveset trisodium: comparison to gadopentetate dimeglumine. Invest Radiol 2007;42:659–64.

25. Casey W, Chew RT, Rebecca AM, et al. Advantages of preoperative computed tomography in deep inferior epigastric artery perforator flap breast reconstruction. Plast Reconstr Surg 2009;123(4): 1148–55.

Dynamic Infrared Thermography

Louis de Weerd, MD, PhD[a],*, James B. Mercer, PhD[b,c],
Sven Weum, MD[b,c]

KEYWORDS

- Perforator flap surgery • Dynamic infrared thermography
- Breast reconstruction • Free flap perfusion • Flap planning
- Skin temperature

Humans are homeotherms, meaning that they are capable of maintaining a constant temperature that is different from that of the surroundings. This is achieved by keeping a fine balance between heat production and heat loss. The necessary heat to keep this constant temperature is generated by metabolism and muscle contraction. Heat is transported through the body with blood acting as the heat transfer medium. The skin plays an important role in the body's temperature regulation. Heat loss to the surroundings is possible by conduction, convection, evaporation, and radiation (**Fig. 1**).[1–3] Under stable ambient conditions of 18°C to 25°C, the principal mechanism to achieve equilibrium between the body and the environment is by radiative heat loss from the skin to the environment. This radiative heat loss takes place in the form of infrared (IR) radiation.[4]

Skin temperature has been used for centuries as an indicator of the physiologic condition and as an indication of possible pathology.[5] There is a defined relationship between the skin temperature and the emitted infrared (IR) radiation from the skin surface.[6] In medical IR thermography, images are produced of a patient's surface temperature based on the IR radiation from the skin.[1,2] Studies in humans have shown that there is a good correlation between skin perfusion and skin temperature. Measurement of skin

temperature can therefore provide indirect information on skin perfusion.[7–10]

The first report on the clinical use of IR thermography as a diagnostic aid came in 1956 when Lawson discovered that the skin temperature over a cancer in a breast was higher than that of normal tissue.[11] He also showed that the venous blood draining the cancer is often warmer than its arterial supply. From then on there has been interest in the clinical use of IR thermography. The technique does not entail the use of ionizing radiation, venous infusion, or invasive procedures. In addition, the technique is easy to perform and images are relatively easy to interpret.

The low sensitivity of early IR cameras made them unsuitable for detecting subtle changes in temperature. Improved IR camera technology with greatly improved temperature sensitivity (<0.1°C) and computer image analysis have led to a resurgence of interest in the applications of medical IR thermography.[1,6] Modern imaging systems offer real-time digital image capture in combination with state-of-the-art computer-assisted image analysis. In these systems, the thermal images are gray scale temperature coded. It is usual to apply additional color coding, with different temperatures being represented by different colors, which greatly helps in interpreting images. The rainbow palette is a frequently used color coding in medical IR thermography with the

Final Disclosure: The authors have nothing to disclose.
[a] Department of Plastic Surgery and Hand Surgery, University Hospital North Norway, N-9038 Tromsø, Norway
[b] Cardiovascular Research Group, Department of Medical Biology, Faculty of Health Sciences, University of Tromsø, N-9037 Tromsø, Norway
[c] Department of Radiology, University Hospital North Norway, N-9038 Tromsø, Norway
* Corresponding author.
E-mail address: louis.de.weerd@unn.no

Clin Plastic Surg 38 (2011) 277–292
doi:10.1016/j.cps.2011.03.013
0094-1298/11/$ – see front matter © 2011 Elsevier Inc. All rights reserved

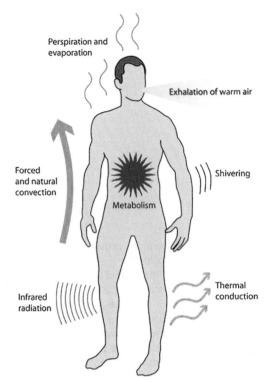

Fig. 1. The body keeps a constant temperature by balancing heat production and heat loss. The illustration shows the main mechanisms involved.

red end of the scale representing warm temperatures and the blue end representing colder temperatures (**Fig. 2**). IR thermography is now used in major fields of medicine, including neurology, rheumatology, dermatology, oncology, and surgery.[1,2,6] In free-flap surgery, the perfusion and reperfusion of the flap are crucial for successful surgery. It is therefore surprising that the use of

IR thermography in flap surgery is so scarcely reported in the literature.

In static IR thermography, a single image is taken. The interpretation of such an image mainly depends on identifying the distribution of hot and cold spots and asymmetric temperature distribution. One of the assumptions when using this method in clinical medicine is that the distribution of body surface temperature is basically symmetric between the left and right sides of the body.[1,4,6]

Because of the interference from complex vascular patterns, it has been proposed to monitor the thermal recovery process after exposure of the area of interest to thermal stress.[12] This technique is called dynamic IR thermography (DIRT). Thermal stress can be achieved by, for example, fan cooling or water immersion, and by applying cold or warm objects to the skin surface. The rate and pattern at which the skin temperature recovers toward its equilibrium is registered with an IR camera.[3,12] **Fig. 3** illustrates the rewarming of the lower abdomen after 2 minutes of fan cooling. A special form of DIRT is the perfusion of tissue with warm or cold perfusate, as for example in organ transplantation and cardiac surgery.[13,14]

In this article, we illustrate how DIRT can provide the plastic surgeon with valuable information in autologous breast reconstruction with the deep inferior epigastric perforator (DIEP) flap.

THE USE OF DIRT IN BREAST RECONSTRUCTION WITH A FREE DIEP FLAP

Breast reconstruction with a free DIEP flap has become increasingly popular in autologous breast reconstruction.[15,16] This flap can provide a large

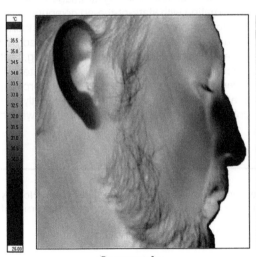

Gray scale

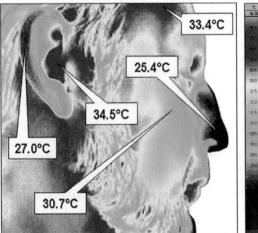

Rainbow palette

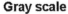

Fig. 2. Two infrared thermograms, the left in gray scale and the right in the rainbow palette.

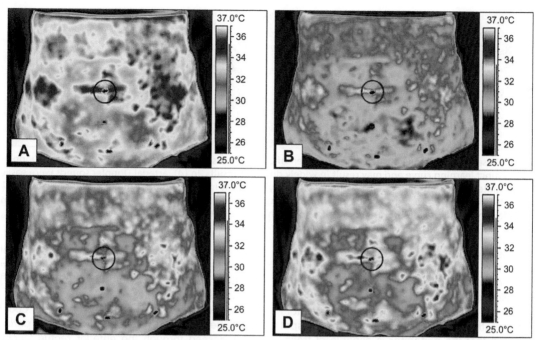

Fig. 3. An illustration of DIRT. The IR thermograms show the lower abdomen in one individual before (*A*), immediately after (*B*), and at 1 (*C*) and 3 minutes (*D*) recovery after a 2-minute period of convective cooling with a desktop fan. The black circles indicate the location of the navel.

quantity of tissue with excellent texture and skin color that allows for the reconstruction of an aesthetically pleasing breast with little donor site morbidity. The disadvantages of using this flap are largely related to the distinct learning curve.[16,17] Adequate preoperative planning, meticulous surgical technique, and a thorough understanding of the vascular anatomy are crucial for a successful postoperative result. Partial and total flap losses owing to inadequate perfusion of the flap are complications that may occur when using this technique, especially by the inexperienced surgeon. Breast reconstruction with a DIEP flap can be divided into 3 phases: a preoperative, an intraoperative, and a postoperative phase. The use of DIRT in each phase is highlighted in the following sections.

The Preoperative Phase

An important consideration in the preoperative planning of a DIEP flap is the selection of a suitable perforator.[16] Although intraoperative selection of a perforator is possible, the large variability in the size and position of the perforators makes this rather complex. Preoperative mapping of the perforators allows the flap to be designed over a dominant perforator and may reduce operative time. Localization of the perforator is considered at least as important as determining its size. It

has been advised to harvest a dominant perforator that is localized closest to the center of the skin flap.[18]

Itoh and Arai[19] illustrated with 2 clinical cases that a perforator flap could be based on the perforator that was identified by the location of a hot spot on the thermal image during the rewarming of the skin after a cold challenge. In 2009, we reported on the value of the use of DIRT in the preoperative planning of the DIEP flap.[20] After the outline of the flap had been drawn on the lower abdomen, the locations of arterial Doppler sounds were marked on the skin with black dots (**Fig. 4**). All patients were examined in a special examination room with a room temperature of 22°C to 24°C and constant humidity and air circulation. Typically, the exposed abdomen was subjected to an acclimatization period at room temperature before the DIRT examination. A desktop fan was used to deliver the cold challenge by blowing air at room temperature over the abdomen for 2 minutes. This cold challenge causes visible changes in skin temperature that are well within the physiologic range, and has a short recovery period of approximately 5 minutes. The results from the analysis of the DIRT examination for each individual patient revealed large variability in the number and positions of hot spots between the left and right side. There was also large variability in the number and positions of hot spots among

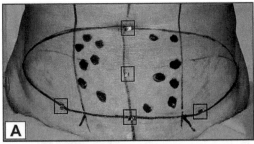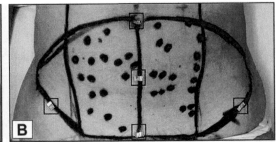

Fig. 4. These 2 photographs of the lower abdomen of 2 individuals illustrate that the use of handheld Doppler has a distinct learning curve and may result in widely different results. In (*A*), arterial Doppler sounds were easily differentiated based on their audible volume with only the most intense Doppler sounds being marked (*black spots*). However, in (*B*), a high number of Doppler sounds were registered all being of similar intensity. This example serves to illustrate the usefulness of finding another technique for locating suitable perforators.

patients (**Fig. 5**). Analysis of the rate and pattern of rewarming of the hot spots allowed a qualitative assessment of all the perforators at the same time. Hot spots that showed rapid and progressive rewarming could be related to suitable perforators intraoperatively. A rapid rewarming at the hot spot indicates that the perforator is capable of transporting more blood to the skin surface than a hot spot with a low rate of rewarming. A rapid progression of rewarming at the hot spot suggests a better-developed vascular network around the hotspot. It appeared that whereas all first-appearing hot spots could be associated with the location of an arterial Doppler sound, not all arterial Doppler sound locations could be related

to a hot spot. In addition, the selected hot spot correlated well with a suitable perforator seen on multidetector row computed tomography (MDCT) scans (**Figs. 6** and **7**).

The location of the hot spot on the skin could easily be related to the location where the perforator passed through the anterior rectus fascia, although the hot spot as well as the associated Doppler sound were slightly more laterally positioned. The more laterally positioned Doppler sounds and hot spots are caused by the lateral course of vessels supplying the skin, as shown by the eminent surgeon and anatomist John Hunter (1728–1793). He explained that the orientation of vessels was a product of differential growth

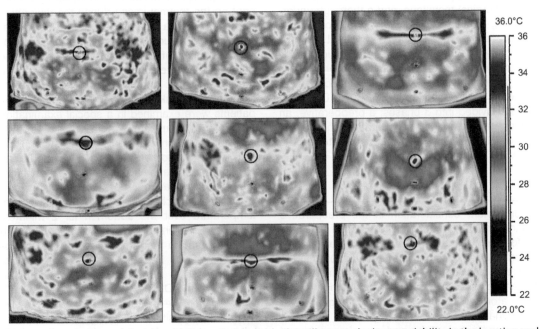

Fig. 5. IR thermograms of the lower abdomen in 9 individuals to illustrate the large variability in the location and intensity of hot spots. Note the asymmetric distribution in each individual.

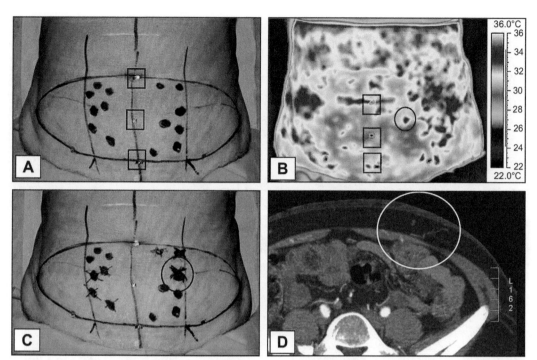

Fig. 6. The flap is outlined on the lower abdomen (*A*). The black dots represent the locations where arterial Doppler sounds were registered. Small pieces of metal tape were used as reference marks (*black squares* in *A* and *B*). The IR thermogram (*B*) was taken 3 minutes after 2 minutes of fan cooling. The black circle indicates the first-appearing hot spot. In (*C*), locations of arterial sounds associated with hot spots are marked with an "X." The selected perforator is marked with a circle and correlates with a suitable perforator on the MDCT scan (*white circle* in *D*).

that had occurred in that area from the stage of fetus to adulthood.[21] Giunta and colleagues[22] found that the preoperative Doppler location on the skin was located within an average distance of 0.8 cm from that of the exit point of the perforator through the fascia. Interestingly, in our study the selected hot spot on the DIRT images was always associated with an audible Doppler sound and a suitable perforator.

The easiest dissection is reported for those perforators that have a perpendicular penetration pattern through the fascia and a short intramuscular course.[18,23] Perforators that are located at the tendinous intersection have these characteristics and are reported to be larger than average.[18,23] Interestingly, these perforators were easily identified with DIRT. The short course of the perforator from the source vessel to the skin explains the rapid rewarming of the skin at the hot spot (**Fig. 8**). In our series of 8 patients who had an additional preoperative MDCT scan, all the perforators as selected from the DIRT examinations could be related to a clearly visible perforator on the MDCT scan. In 6 of these patients, the selected perforator was located at the tendinous intersection. The results of the DIRT

examinations showed a different rate and pattern of rewarming for DIEP and superficial inferior epigastric artery (SIEA) flaps. Although the number of SIEA flaps in our series was small, it appeared that if the SIEA system was dominant, only small hot spots were seen at the center of the lower abdomen in contrast to the situation where the deep inferior epigastric artery (DIEA) system was dominant. The more laterally positioned vascular territory of the SIEA flap, as well as the different vascular anatomy, help to explain the differences in the results obtained from the DIRT examinations of DIEP and SIEA flaps. To reduce donor site morbidity, surgeons may follow the algorithm as proposed by Arnež and colleagues[24] and explore the possible use of an SIEA flap before they decide to harvest a DIEP flap. Using this algorithm, one can rule out the existence of a dominant SIEA system before one uses the results of the DIRT examination for a DIEP flap.

The Use of DIRT in the Intraoperative Phase

The intraoperative phase of breast reconstruction with a DIEP flap can be divided into 3 periods: the period of dissection of the perforator, the

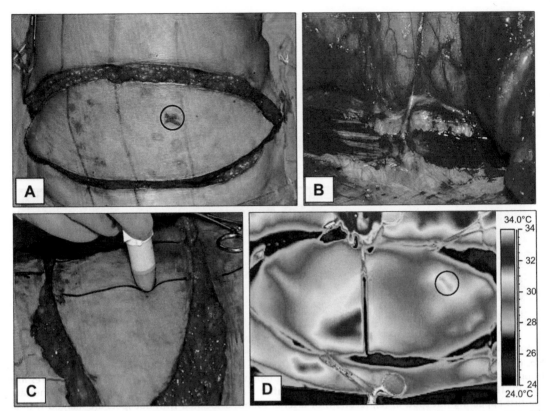

Fig. 7. Intraoperatively, the selected perforator (*A*) coincided with a perforator at the tendinous intersection (*B*). After the perforator was dissected free, its location can be still registered as an arterial Doppler sound (*C*) as well as a hot spot in the IR thermogram (*black circle* in *D*). In the IR thermogram the midline is indicated, the contralateral side has, at this point, not been dissected.

period after opening of the anastomoses, and the period of flap modeling and inset.

One of the disadvantages of perforator flap surgery is the complex dissection of perforators. A meticulous microsurgical technique is required to avoid inadvertent damage to the perforator. In 2006, we reported on the intraoperative use of DIRT in free DIEP flap surgery.[25] After the selected perforator is dissected and with the flap still at the lower abdomen, DIRT can be used to confirm patency of the perforator. Normally a hot spot will be seen on the IR images that correlates with the location of the entrance point of the perforator into the flap. The quality of the perforator can be assessed by analyzing the rate and pattern of rewarming after the skin area above the perforator is exposed to a conductive thermal challenge. A metal plate at room temperature is gently applied to the skin surface for 30 seconds (**Figs. 9** and **10**).

A rapid and pronounced rewarming at the hot spot confirms that the perforator has not been damaged during dissection. In case there is no rewarming or poor rewarming, the surgeon can decide to harvest another suitable perforator.

Although the perforator can also be checked by using a handheld Doppler probe, in our experience the registration of an audible arterial Doppler sound was always registered later than the rewarming seen on the IR images. After the flap is dissected free and the pedicle to the flap is ligated and cut, the DIEP flap is ready for transfer to the thoracic wall. With cessation of the blood supply to the flap, the period of primary ischemia starts. As there is no perfusion, the flap cools down.

A second critical part in the intraoperative procedure is the anastomosis of the donor vessels to the recipient vessels on the thoracic wall. It is especially the period immediately after completion of the microsurgical anastomoses that is considered important. Thrombosis at the vascular anastomosis has been implicated as the main reason for flap loss.[26] Experimental studies have shown that formation of an arterial thrombus following release of the clamps reaches a maximum after 15 minutes. After 30 minutes, most of the thrombus has been lysed.[27] Recently, Wolff and colleagues[28] evaluated the incidence and time of intraoperative complications in head and neck

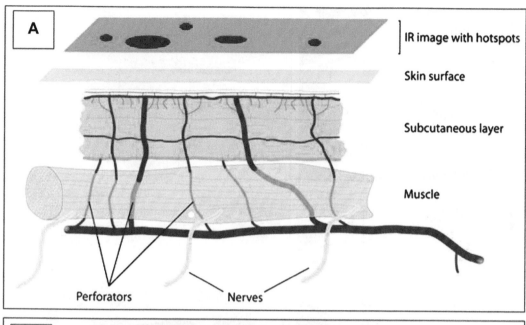

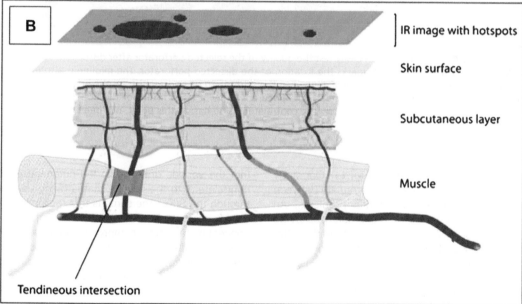

Fig. 8. This figure illustrates how direct perforators with a short intramuscular course may be associated with a bright hot spot (*A*). Direct perforators at the tendinous intersection have a short intramuscular course and have a larger than average caliber and show up as bright hot spots (*B*).

microsurgery. Based on their results, they concluded that the microvascular anastomosis should be controlled for at least 45 minutes before wound closure. Just before opening of the anastomoses, flap temperature is at its lowest and IR thermal images of the skin surface are diffuse without clear patterns. By opening the anastomosis, the flap becomes reperfused with blood.

The rate and pattern of rewarming is registered with the IR camera. The rapid (often within seconds) appearance of a hot spot clearly indicates where the rewarming of the flap starts. A progressive increase in skin surface temperature of the flap becomes visible. In the area around the first-appearing hot spot, other hot spots appear with time, the number and pattern varying

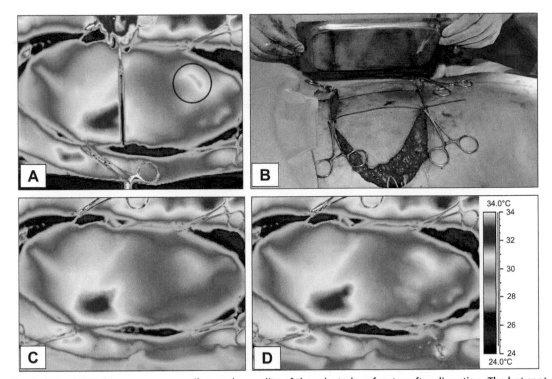

Fig. 9. Using DIRT, the surgeon can easily test the quality of the selected perforator after dissection. The hot spot (*circle*) on the IR thermogram (*A*) marks the location of the dissected perforator. The midline is also indicated. A metal plate (*B*) at room temperature is applied to the skin for 30 seconds, which results in a mild conductive cooling (*C*). Note that the hot spot has nearly disappeared. In (*D*), a rapid return of the hot spot after cooling indicates perfusion through the perforator. The contralateral side has, at this point, not been dissected.

greatly from patient to patient (**Fig. 11**). Our study showed that it is possible to differentiate between arterial and venous anastomotic problems. An arterial anastomotic failure is characterized by no rewarming or by a cooling down of the flap after an initial period of rewarming. For a venous anastomotic failure, the IR images show diffuse rewarming with no individual hot spots. Warm blood enters, but cannot leave the flap. Tenorio and colleagues[29] also showed in an experimental study the usefulness of intraoperative DIRT in detecting occlusion of the arterial and venous pedicle.

In DIEP flaps that included tissue from the contralateral side of the midline, an additional venous drainage route using the contralateral superficial inferior epigastric vein (SIEV) resulted in an improved overall rewarming of the flap that is easily documentable with IR thermography. The SIEV may be used as a "life boat" in case of venous congestion of the DIEP flap.[30] An anatomic study on the venous drainage of the transverse rectus abdominis musculocutaneous (TRAM) flap by Carramenha e Costa and colleagues[31] showed

that the venous drainage of the cutaneous part, contralateral to the muscle that is being used, is through the SIEV. The same is true for the DIEP.

In flaps that showed clinical signs of venous congestion, a dramatic improvement in skin color was seen after opening of a second route for venous drainage. Opening of a second route for venous drainage was associated with an improved rate and pattern of rewarming (**Fig. 12**). The changes seen on the IR images always preceded the clinical signs of improved perfusion. It is likely that an increase in venous drainage results in better reperfusion of the flap.[32]

During the intraoperative period of flap modeling and flap inset, circulation problems may occur because of external compression or torsion of the pedicle. In perforator flaps, where the pedicle to the flap is not protected by a muscle cuff, as in myocutaneous flaps, external compression and torsion of the pedicle occur more commonly.[33] Reperfusion problems because of external compression or torsion may eventually lead to a secondary thrombosis postoperatively. DIRT has shown to be able to detect these reperfusion

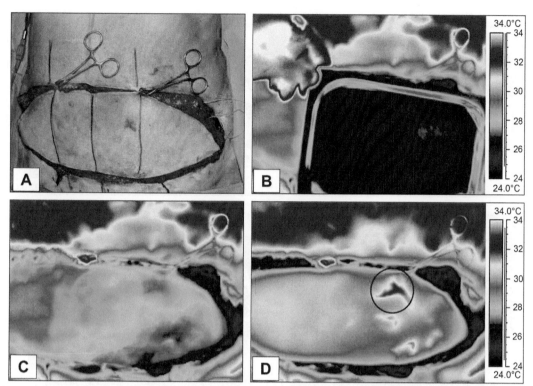

Fig. 10. The same flap as in **Fig. 9** following completion of dissection of the contralateral side. The whole flap (*A*) now depends on its perfusion through the selected perforator. The IR thermogram in (*B*) shows a conductive cold challenge being applied with a metal plate at room temperature. The cooling effect and the disappearance of hot spots can be seen in (*C*). Rewarming starts at the bright hot spot (*circle*) (*D*) that is positioned over the perforator location. The number of hot spots has also increased, indicating the existence of a well-developed vascular network.

problems both intraoperatively as well as at the end of the operation.[25] Intraoperatively this can be seen as a rapid disappearance of the hot spot pattern with the thermal distribution pattern becoming more diffuse. Perfusion of the flap can be easily checked with DIRT at any stage during or after the operation. All the surgeon has to do is to analyze the rate and pattern of rewarming of the flap after the skin surface has been exposed to a conductive cold challenge with a metal plate at room temperature that is gently brought in contact with the skin (**Fig. 13**).

The Postoperative Use of DIRT

During the postoperative phase, the flap is closely monitored for signs of compromised perfusion. Although free tissue transfer has become a well-established technique in reconstructive surgery with high success rates, complications related to problems with the vascular anastomosis do occur. The most critical postoperative period for anasto-motic failure in free-flap surgery seems to be the first 24 hours after surgery.[34] Successful outcomes of explorations are reported to be inversely related

to the time interval between the onset of ischemia and its recognition.[35] Most surgeons rely on clinical observation of skin perfusion using subjective signs, such as skin color, capillary refill, skin temperature, and turgor. Temperature measurement of skin flaps during the postoperative phase is one of the oldest monitoring methods of free flaps and is often included in the protocols of postoperative monitoring of flaps.

The postoperative phase will also highlight whether flap design has been optimal. Current flap design is based on the angiosome concept by Taylor and Palmer[21]: the stepwise progressive perfusion of vascular territories and the tenet that a viable flap can safely include the angiosome of the source artery and one immediately adjacent angiosome. Necrosis tends to occur in the next or subsequent angiosome. The surgeon has, however, no exact information about the size of the angiosomes. In fact, angiosomes can vary considerably in size and position as, for example, is the case on the lower abdomen.[21] Imbalance between perfusion and flap size may, even with perfect arterial and venous anastomoses, lead to partial flap failure. Monitoring the flap can provide

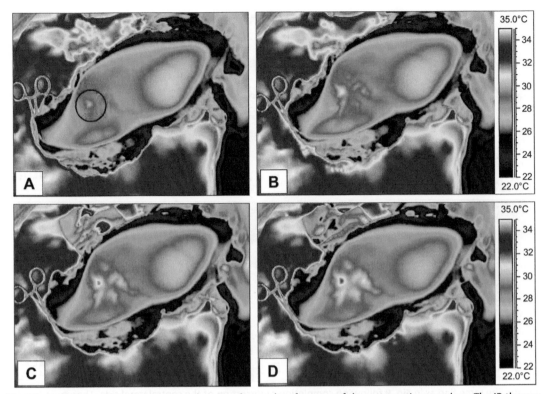

Fig. 11. A sequence of IR thermograms showing the results of a successful anastomotic procedure. The IR thermogram in (*A*) was taken only a few seconds after the anastomoses had been opened. Note the rapid appearance of a hot spot (circled in *A*). Not only does this hot spot rapidly become warmer but note also the appearance of other hot spots within the same area (*B–D*). The contralateral side of the flap shows a diffuse area that is warm but cools down over time. This is an artifact caused by an external heat source (microscope lamp).

the surgeon with valuable information that may help to improve her or his understanding of flap perfusion and design.

We reported on the postoperative use of DIRT in breast reconstruction with a DIEP flap.[36] After an acclimatization period in a special examination room, the uncovered reconstructed breast was exposed to a thermal cold challenge for 2 minutes using a desktop fan. The rate and pattern of rewarming were registered with an IR camera. The results showed that the perfusion of a DIEP flap is a dynamic process with a stepwise progression during the first postoperative week. The stepwise progression of perfusion of the abdominoplasty flap was already reported by Scheflan and Dinner in 1983 for the pedicled TRAM flap.[37] They divided the flap into 4 equal parts and numbered them according to their clinical impression of perfusion during surgery. The quality of perfusion becomes poorer as the zone number increases. The 4 zones are actually an adaptation of the angiosomes of the superficial and deep epigastric arterial systems as described by Taylor and Palmer.[21] Angiosomes throughout the body are usually interconnected to adjacent angiosomes at every

tissue level by reduced-caliber choke vessels, but sometimes by true anastomoses.

The most interesting finding of our study is that there is a stepwise progression in the perfusion of the DIEP flap at 2 levels: the subdermal level and the subcutaneous level, each with its own time sequence (**Fig. 14**). A plausible explanation can be found in the anatomic studies by among others Taylor and Palmer[21] and El-Mrakby and Milner.[38,39] The DIEP flap receives its blood supply through a direct perforator. This perforator has a direct course to the skin where it connects with the subdermal plexus. After the anastomoses had been opened, a bright hot spot could be seen that was positioned over the entrance point of the perforator in the flap. The skin surface showed a rapid increase in temperature that started in zone I at the hot spot. This was followed by the adjacent zone on the ipsilateral side, then the adjacent zone across the midline, and finally the contralateral zone IV. During subsequent days, there was an increase in the number of hot spots on the IR images. Hot spots were initially confined to zone I, but were seen on day 1 also in the adjacent ipsilateral zone. For most flaps,

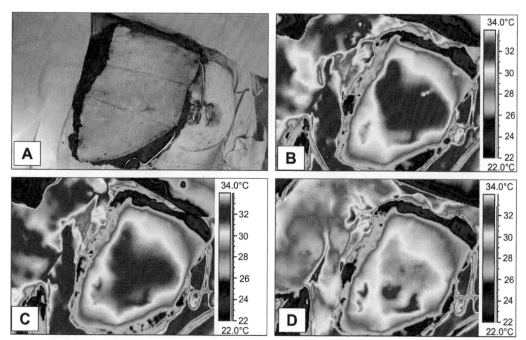

Fig. 12. A sequence of IR thermograms of a DIEP flap (A) showing venous congestion after a successful anasto-motic procedure. The venous congestion is indicated by the fact that the flap has become diffusely warm (B). Following a second venous anastomosis, this congestion is relieved within seconds. Accumulated warm blood is removed from the flap and the pattern of hot spots reappears (C and D).

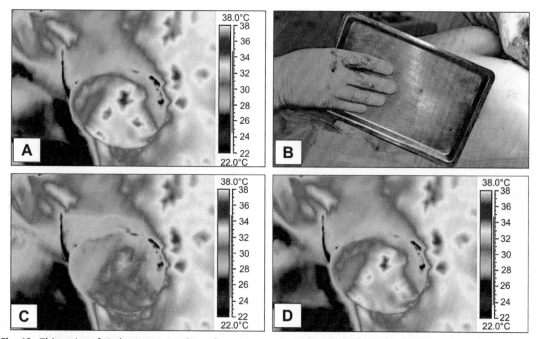

Fig. 13. This series of IR thermograms shows how DIRT at the end of the operation can be used to confirm perfu-sion of a DIEP flap through its perforator. The thermogram in (A) shows the DIEP flap before a mild conductive cooling of the skin by using a metal plate (B). The effect of the cooling is seen in (C) and the very rapid return of hot spots in (D) confirms perfusion of the flap.

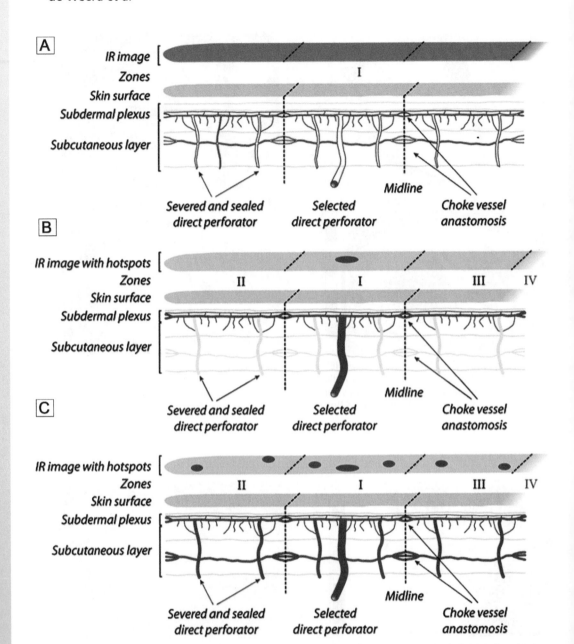

Fig. 14. This figure illustrates the stepwise progression of perfusion of a DIEP flap at the subdermal and subcutaneous level. In (A), the flap is not perfused and the skin surface in the IR thermogram will appear cold and without any hotspots. The subdermal plexus will be perfused through the selected perforator (B). A hot spot will appear over the entrance point of the perforator in the flap. From here the skin will become rewarmed in a stepwise fashion. First zone I rewarms followed by the adjacent ipsilateral zone II and finally zones III and IV across the midline. (C) The subcutaneous tissue will also be perfused in a stepwise fashion in the same order. The rewarming pattern with additional hot spots is explained by the perfusion of other direct perforators after interconnections with the selected direct perforator in zone I have opened. Choke vessels are located between zones in the subdermal plexus.

hot spots began to appear across the midline on day 3 and their number increased on day 6 (**Fig. 15**). The sequence of rewarming of the zones is for both levels similar to that found by Holm and colleagues[40] for the DIEP flap.

Although the order of rewarming of the zones is the same at the subdermal and subcutaneous levels, there is a difference in the time sequence. The results suggest that the choke vessels at the subdermal level cause less resistance to

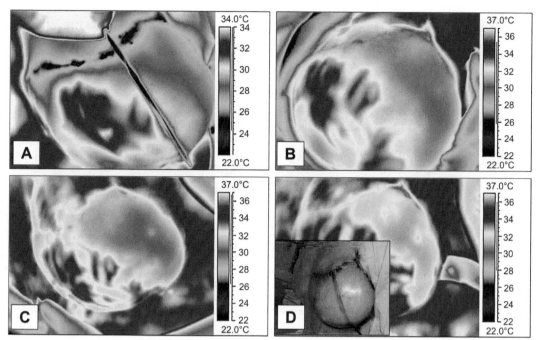

Fig. 15. A sequence of IR thermograms showing the evolution of perfusion in the days following a DIEP operation. In the IR thermogram taken at the end of the operation (*A*), the midline is indicated with a surgical instrument (*blue line*). Note that the flap on the contralateral side is warm (*A*) but without visible hotspots. This pattern is similar on day 1 after the operation (*B*). However, vague hotspots begin to appear on day 3 (*C*) and become clearly visible on the sixth postoperative day (*D*). These new-appearing hot spots are also associated with an arterial Doppler sound.

circulation compared with those at the subcutaneous level. Adequate perfusion of the zones at the subdermal level of the free DIEP flaps is therefore reached earlier than at the subcutaneous level. With the stepwise opening of the choke vessels between the angiosomes, perforators located in adjacent angiosomes become perfused. The perfusion of these perforators became visible as hot spots. The hot spots at the contralateral side appeared 1 or 2 days after the hot spots had appeared on the ipsilateral side. This phenomenon cannot be explained by angiogenesis because of the short time elapsed.

It has been reported that flaps have a period of hyperemia during the first postoperative days.[41] In our study, the hyperemia was initially seen on the whole flap and most in zone I. During subsequent days, a decrease in hyperemia was registered that coincided with an increase in the number of hot spots on the contralateral side. Although the hot spots on the contralateral side became more visible on consecutive examination days, the rate of rewarming of hot spots on the ipsilateral side decreased. Such can be explained by a redistribution of blood within the whole flap that takes place because of an increase in the diameter of choke vessel lumen in the subcutaneous tissue. As a result, the perfusion of the

subcutaneous tissue improves, especially on the contralateral side and the hyperemia subsides.

Some articles report that nearly the entire transverse abdominal flap can be harvested as a DIEP flap.[42,43] Others report that only 70% of the transverse abdominal flap can be safely used as a DIEP flap.[44] From earlier studies, it is known that the subdermal plexus contributes to the perfusion of the superficial subcutaneous layer. In a cross-sectional radiographic study, Taylor[45] revealed a blood supply to the superficial subcutaneous layer caused by "raining down" from the subdermal plexus. In their experimental study, Schaverien and colleagues[46] found a similar result. This might explain why skin and superficial subcutaneous fat may survive in the presence of fat necrosis in the deep subcutaneous layer. This deep layer becomes adequately perfused only after choke vessels in the subcutaneous layer have dilated. This might also explain why nearly the entire transverse abdominal flap can be safely used if this flap is thin. As commented by Nahabedian,[47] not only the size of the DIEP flap but also its volume has to be taken into consideration.

The analyses of our results indicate that the perfusion of DIEP flap shows great similarity with the processes that occur during flap delay in animal studies. These animal studies show

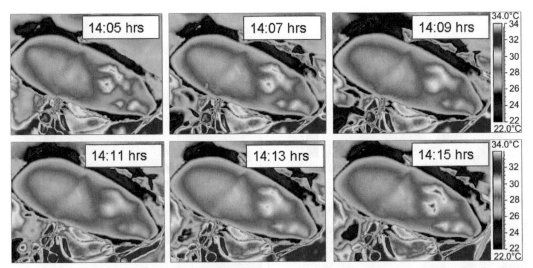

Fig. 16. This sequence of IR thermograms of a DIEP flap following successful anastomoses to the internal mammary vessels is presented to show that DIRT is able to provide the surgeon with real-time feedback on the physiology of flap perfusion. In the middle of the 10-minute period depicted by this series of thermograms, the bright hot spots begin to disappear. This was caused by a fall in blood pressure. With restoration of blood pressure, the hot spots returned.

a progressive sequential dilatation of choke vessels that was most dramatic between 48 and 72 hours after surgery.[48,49] Dhar and Taylor[48] stated that the time sequence for delay appears to be similar in different species and in different tissues, suggesting the possibility of a universal process for delay. Our results suggest that the choke vessels at the subdermal level cause less resistance to circulation compared with those at the subcutaneous level. A possible explanation for this may be related to the function of the skin in the body's temperature regulation. Recently, Busic and Das-Gupta[50] criticized the use of temperature measurement in the monitoring of DIEP flaps. The postoperative use of DIRT in breast reconstruction with a DIEP flap showed that the temperature differed from location to location and that the temperature changed over time. Absolute temperature measurements are perhaps less informative than the information on the rate and pattern of rewarming obtained with DIRT.

SUMMARY

The use of DIRT in breast reconstruction with a DIEP flap can provide the surgeon with valuable information in the preoperative, intraoperative, and postoperative phases. In the preoperative planning of perforator flaps, the use of MDCT angiography has become the gold standard in some hospitals.[51,52] The high spatial and temporal resolution achieved with MDCT angiography allows for a precise description of the origin, intramuscular course, and point of

fascia penetration of the perforator. Although DIRT does not show the morphology of the perforators, it identifies suitable perforators based on the perforators' physiology. To adopt MDCT as a routine preoperative imaging modality, the benefit to the patient, for both the reconstructed breast and the abdominal donor site, must outweigh the problems associated with the procedure. These include the risk of intravenous contrast injection, exposure to ionizing radiation, and associated cost. Recent literature cautions against the rising exposure of ionizing radiation to the population from computed tomography (CT) examinations.[53,54] IR thermography has none of these disadvantages. The intraoperative use of DIRT seems self-evident. The technique allows assessment of perfusion and reperfusion in real time and thus provides the surgeon immediate feedback. The surgeon can take corrective action when it is most effective. In open heart surgery, neurosurgery, and organ transplant surgery, DIRT provides the surgeon with valuable information on perfusion and reperfusion of the organs.[13,14,55] Surprisingly, reports on intraoperative use of DIRT were limited to a few articles, such as those published by Salmi and colleagues[41] and Wolff and colleagues.[56] The use of DIRT in the postoperative phase shows that the perfusion of the DIEP flap is a dynamic process with a stepwise progression at the subdermal level and the subcutaneous level, each with its own time sequence. Such information may help to improve flap design and reduce therewith the risk of partial flap failure owing to an imbalance between flap geometry and flap perfusion.

The information obtained from DIRT examinations can be of great value to the plastic surgeon in perforator flap surgery. DIRT provides, however, information only on the physiology of the perforator and not on its morphology. It is therefore important that the surgeon has a thorough knowledge on the flap's vascular anatomy and physiology when interpreting the results obtained from DIRT (**Fig. 16**).

ACKNOWLEDGMENTS

The authors thank Mr Rod Wolstenholme, Audiovisual Department, Faculty of Health Sciences, University of Tromsø, Tromsø, Norway, for his technical assistance in preparing Figures 8 and 14.

REFERENCES

1. Jiang LJ, Ng EY, Yeo AC, et al. A perspective on medical infrared imaging. J Med Eng Technol 2005;29:257–67.
2. Jones BF, Plassmann P. Digital infrared thermal imaging of human skin. IEEE Eng Med Biol Mag 2002;21:41–8.
3. Pascoe DD, Mercer JB, de Weerd L. Physiology of thermal signals. In: Diakides NA, Bronzino JD, editors. Medical infrared imaging. Boca Raton (FL): CRC Press, Taylor & Francis Group; 2008. p. 6-1–6-20.
4. Ammer K, Ring FE. Standard procedures for infrared imaging in medicine. In: Diakides NA, Bronzino JD, editors. Medical infrared imaging. Boca Raton (FL): CRC Press, Taylor & Francis Group; 2008. p. 22-1–22-9.
5. Ring FE, Jones BF. The historical development of thermometry and thermal imaging in medicine. In: Diakides NA, Bronzino JD, editors. Medical infrared imaging. Boca Raton (FL): CRC Press, Taylor & Francis Group; 2008. p. 2-1–2-5.
6. Jones BF. A reappraisal of the use of infrared thermal image analysis in medicine. IEEE Trans Med Imaging 1998;17:1019–27.
7. Francis JE, Roggli R, Love TJ, et al. Thermography as a means of blood perfusion measurements. J Biomech Eng 1979;101:246–9.
8. Awwad AM, White RJ, Webster MH, et al. The effect of temperature on blood flow in island and free skin flaps: an experimental study. Br J Plast Surg 1983; 36:373–82.
9. Mercer JB, de Weerd L. The effect of water-filtered infrared (IR)-A (wIRA) irradiation on skin temperature and skin blood flow as evaluated by infrared thermography and scanning laser Doppler imaging. Thermol Int 2005;15:89–94.
10. Merla A, Di Romualdo S, Di Donato L, et al. Combined thermal and laser Doppler imaging in the assessment of cutaneous tissue perfusion. Conf Proc IEEE Eng Med Biol Soc 2007;2007:2630–3.
11. Lawson RN. Implications of surface temperatures in the diagnosis of breast cancer. Can Med Assoc J 1956;75:309–11.
12. Wilson SB, Spence VA. Dynamic thermography imaging method for quantifying dermal perfusion: potential and limitations. Med Biol Eng Comput 1989;27:496–501.
13. Iwahashi H, Tashiro T, Morishige N, et al. New method of thermal coronary angiography for intraoperative patency control in off-pump and on-pump coronary artery bypass grafting. Ann Thorac Surg 2007;84:1504–7.
14. Pabisiak K, Romanowski M, Myslak M, et al. Variations in temperature of the donor kidney during cold ischemia time and subsequent assessment of reperfusion using the application of thermovision camera. Transplant Proc 2003;35:2157–9.
15. Blondeel PN. Soft tissue reconstruction with perforator flaps. In: Siemionow MZ, editor. Tissue surgery. Singapore: Springer-Verlag London Limited; 2006. p. 87–100.
16. Granzow JW, Levine JL, Chiu ES, et al. Breast reconstruction using perforator flaps. J Surg Oncol 2006; 94:441–54.
17. Busic V, Das-Gupta R, Mesic H, et al. The deep inferior epigastric perforator flap for breast reconstruction, the learning curve explored. J Plast Reconstr Aesthet Surg 2006;59:580–4.
18. Blondeel PN, Neligan PC. Complications: avoidance and treatment. In: Blondeel PN, Morris SF, Hallock GC, et al, editors. Perforator flaps. Anatomy, technique, and clinical applications. St Louis (MO): Quality Medical Publishing, Inc; 2008. p. 116–28.
19. Itoh Y, Arai K. The deep inferior epigastric artery free skin flap: anatomic study and clinical application. Plast Reconstr Surg 1993;91:853–63.
20. de Weerd L, Weum S, Mercer JB. The value of dynamic infrared thermography (DIRT) in perforator selection and planning of DIEP flaps. Ann Plast Surg 2009;63:274–9.
21. Taylor GI, Palmer JH. The vascular territories (angiosomes) of the body: experimental study and clinical applications. Br J Plast Surg 1987;40:113–41.
22. Giunta RE, Geisweid A, Feller AM. The value of preoperative Doppler sonography for planning free perforator flaps. Plast Reconstr Surg 2000;105: 2381–6.
23. Blondeel PN. One hundred free DIEP flap breast reconstructions: a personal experience. Br J Plast Surg 1999;52:104–11.
24. Arnež ZM, Khan U, Pogorelec D, et al. Rational selection of flaps from the abdomen in breast reconstruction to reduce donor site morbidity. Br J Plast Surg 1999;52:351–4.
25. de Weerd L, Mercer JB, Bøe Setså L. Intraoperative dynamic infrared thermography and free-flap surgery. Ann Plast Surg 2006;57:279–84.

26. Panchapakesan V, Addison P, Beausang E, et al. Role of thrombolysis in free-flap salvage. J Reconstr Microsurg 2003;19:523–9.

27. Rosenbaum TJ, Sundt TM. Thrombus formation and endothelial alterations in microarterial anastomoses. J Neurosurg 1997;47:430–41.

28. Wolff KD, Hözle F, Wysluch A, et al. Incidence and time of intraoperative vascular complications in head and neck microsurgery. Microsurgery 2008; 28:143–6.

29. Tenorio X, Mahajan AL, Wettstein R, et al. Early detection of flap failure using a new thermographic device. J Surg Res 2009;151:15–21.

30. Wechselberger G, Schoeller T, Bauer T, et al. Venous superdrainage in deep inferior epigastric perforator flap breast reconstruction. Plast Reconstr Surg 2001;108:162–4.

31. Carramenha e Costa MA, Carriquiry C, Vasconez LO, et al. An anatomic study of the venous drainage of the transverse rectus abdominis musculocutaneous flap. Plast Reconstr Surg 1987;79:208–13.

32. Chow SP, Chen DZ, Gu YD. The significance of venous drainage in free flap transfer. Plast Reconstr Surg 1993;91:713–5.

33. Celik N, Wei FC. Technical tips in perforator flap harvest. Clin Plast Surg 2003;30:469–72.

34. Smit JM, Acosta R, Zeebergts CJ, et al. Early reintervention of compromised free flaps improves success rate. Microsurgery 2007;27:612–6.

35. Jones NF. Intraoperative and postoperative monitoring of microsurgical free tissue transfers. Clin Plast Surg 1992;19:783–97.

36. de Weerd L, Miland ÅO, Mercer JB. Perfusion dynamics of free DIEP and SIEA flaps during the first postoperative week monitored with dynamic infrared thermography (DIRT). Ann Plast Surg 2009;62:40–7.

37. Scheflan M, Dinner MI. The transverse abdominal island flap: part II. Surgical technique. Ann Plast Surg 1983;10:120–9.

38. El-Mrakby HH, Milner RH. The vascular anatomy of the lower anterior abdominal wall: a microdissection study on the deep inferior epigastric vessels and the perforator branches. Plast Reconstr Surg 2002;109: 539–43 [discussion by Taylor GI, p. 544–7].

39. El Mrakby HH, Milner RH. Bimodal distribution of the blood supply to lower abdominal fat: histological study of the microcirculation of the lower abdominal wall. Ann Plast Surg 2003;50:165–70.

40. Holm C, Mayr M, Höfter E, et al. Perfusion zones of the DIEP flap revisited: a clinical study. Plast Reconstr Surg 2006;117:37–43.

41. Salmi AM, Tukiainen E, Asko-Seljavaara S. Thermographic mapping of perforators and skin blood flow in the free transverse rectus abdominis musculocutaneous flap. Ann Plast Surg 1995;35: 159–64.

42. Ulusal BG, Cheng MH, Wei FC. Breast reconstruction using the entire transverse abdominal adipocutaneous flap based on unilateral superficial or deep inferior epigastric vessels. Plast Reconstr Surg 2006;117:1395–403.

43. Cheng MH, Robles JA, Ulusal BG, et al. Reliability of zone IV in the deep inferior epigastric perforator flap: a single center's experience with 74 cases. Breast 2006;15:158–66.

44. Kroll SS. Fat necrosis in free transverse rectus abdominis myocutaneous and deep inferior epigastric perforator flaps. Plast Reconstr Surg 2000;106: 576–83.

45. Taylor GI. The vascular anatomy of the lower anterior abdominal wall: a microdissection study on the deep inferior epigastric vessels and the perforator branches. Plast Reconstr Surg 2002;109:544–7 [discussion].

46. Schaverien M, Saint-Cyr M, Arbique G, et al. Arterial and venous anatomies of the DIEP inferior epigastric perforator and superficial inferior epigastric artery flaps. Plast Reconstr Surg 2008;121:1909–19.

47. Nahabedian MY. Breast reconstruction using the entire transverse abdominal adipocutaneous flap based on unilateral superficial or deep inferior epigastric vessels. Plast Reconstr Surg 2006;117: 1404–6 [discussion].

48. Dhar SC, Taylor GI. The delay phenomenon: the story unfolds. Plast Reconstr Surg 1999;104:2079–91.

49. Aydin MA, Mavili ME. Examining microcirculation improves the angiosome theory in explaining the delay phenomenon in a rabbit model. J Reconstr Microsurg 2003;19:187–94.

50. Busic V, Das-Gupta R. Temperature monitoring in free flap surgery. Br J Plast Surg 2004;57:588.

51. Masia J, Clavero JA, Larrañaga JR, et al. Multidetector-row tomography in the planning of abdominal perforator flaps. J Plast Reconstr Aesthet Surg 2006;59:594–9.

52. Rozen WM, Phillips TJ, Ashton MW, et al. Preoperative imaging for DIEA perforator flaps: a comparative study of computed tomographic angiography and Doppler ultrasound. Plast Reconstr Surg 2008;121:9–16.

53. Brenner DJ, Hall EJ. Computed tomography: an increasing source of radiation exposure. N Engl J Med 2007;357:2277–84.

54. Lee CI, Haims AH, Monico EP, et al. Diagnostic CT scans: assessment of patient, physician, and radiologist awareness of radiation dose and possible risks. Radiology 2004;231:393–8.

55. Okada Y, Kawamata T, Kawashima A, et al. Intraoperative application of thermography in extracranial-intracranial bypass surgery. Neurosurgery 2007;60: 362–5.

56. Wolff KD, Telzrow T, Rudolph KH, et al. Isotope perfusion and infrared thermography of arterialised, venous flow-through and pedicled venous flaps. Br J Plast Surg 1995;48:61–70.

Fluorescent Angiography

Michael R. Zenn, MD

KEYWORDS

- Laser angiography • Fluorescent angiography
- Tissue perfusion • Indocyanine green • ICG • SPY

Fluorescent angiography is a simple and effective real-time tool for measurement of tissue perfusion both in and out of the operating room. The technology is based on indocyanine green (ICG) dye that absorbs light in the near-infrared (NIR) spectrum. Advances in technology have allowed the surgeon to use fluorescent angiography in the operating room in real time, under complete control of the surgeon. Although used experimentally in the late 1990s, by the mid 2000s the technology was already in regular use by some plastic surgeons.[1] For the first time, surgeons could immediately see perfusion in the operated tissues multiple times throughout a procedure as needs changed. Most importantly, use of the dye and the laser has been proved to be safe in humans. The true impact of the technology on the understanding of our specialty is only beginning to be felt.

ICG dye is a water-soluble tricarbocyanine dye that was originally developed by the Eastman Kodak company for use in infrared photography. It was introduced into clinical use when, as a token of appreciation for his treatment at the Mayo Clinic, an executive with the Eastman Kodak Company sent a variety of dyes to a clinician who was looking for suitable dyes that could be safely administered to patients and easily measured in blood. The clinically useful formulation of the dye, a stable lyophilized powder, was developed. For a time ICG was referred to as "Fox Green" after the cardiologist Dr Irwin Fox, who was responsible for its introduction into clinical practice. Initially ICG was used to assess cardiac output by means of a dye-dilution technique.[2] It was later also used to assess arteriovenous fistulae[3] and renal blood flow.[4] The observation that ICG is excreted exclusively via the liver led to its use in assessing liver function and blood flow.[5,6] The near-infrared absorption and emission of light by ICG makes it particularly well suited to visualizing small blood vessels. In the early 1970s, Flower developed techniques for acquisition of fluorescence angiograms of the choroid using ICG.[7,8] All current fluorescence imaging using ICG is in essence adaptation of the principles developed by Flower, with the benefit of improvement in NIR-sensitive cameras and light sources.

One of the biggest advantages of ICG over other dyes such as fluorescein is its rapid clearance from the tissues. Following intravascular administration, ICG is rapidly and extensively bound to plasma proteins, with α-lipoproteins being the major carrier in humans.[9] The ICG is thus confined to the intravascular compartment with little leakage into the interstitium, making it an ideal blood pool contrast agent. By contrast, fluorescein remains in the interstitium and therefore can only be used once, and gives no information about dynamic perfusion. The plasma half-life of ICG is very short, approximately 3 to 5 minutes in humans, with the dye being taken up by the liver and being excreted into the bile without any further metabolism.[10] There is no renal excretion of ICG and so there is no contraindication for use in patients with renal insufficiency. Since its introduction into clinical practice, ICG has shown an excellent safety profile with a low incidence of adverse events of about 1 in 42,000 patients. Anaphylactic reactions are rare.

Disclosure: Dr Zenn is a paid consultant for the Novadaq Corporation, maker of the SPY system and LifeCell, distributor of the SPY system.
Division of Plastic and Reconstructive Surgery, Duke University Medical Center, 136 Baker House, Trent Drive, Durham, NC 27710-3358, USA
E-mail address: Michael.Zenn@duke.edu

Clin Plastic Surg 38 (2011) 293–300
doi:10.1016/j.cps.2011.03.009
0094-1298/11/$ – see front matter © 2011 Elsevier Inc. All rights reserved

The ICG contains iodide, so patients sensitive to iodides should undergo have this study. Most reactions if any are usually mild in nature, for example, feeling of warmth or sore throat.[11]

A typical intraoperative imaging system comprises an imaging camera that houses an 806-nm diode laser to provide near-infrared illumination. This low-level laser does not require the use of protective goggles by operating room staff or the operating surgeon. Optics within the camera can provide even NIR illumination over fields as large as 20 × 20 cm or as small as a centimeter in an operating microscope. Cameras have also been adopted for use in robotic surgery and endoscopic surgery. Image sequences are usually captured at 30 frames per second, and the image sequences are displayed on a monitor in real time for the surgeon to assess. Most systems have a computer for further analysis, review, and archival of the data.

The SPY system (Novadaq, Mississauga, ON, USA; Canada/LifeCell, Branchburg, NJ, USA) is the most commonly used system in plastic and reconstructive surgery (**Fig. 1**). It was originally developed for use in coronary artery bypass graft surgery to confirm the patency of bypass grafts and was cleared for this indication in Canada, Europe, and Japan in 2001. Several publications reported that SPY imaging detected nonfunctioning grafts in 4% to 8% of patients, and this finding was consistent across sites and surgical procedures that is, on-pump or off-pump.[12–22] The use of SPY imaging was subsequently expanded to solid organ transplantation including, liver and kidney[23,24] and pancreas.[25] The SPY system received regulatory clearance from the US Food and Drug Administration for use in coronary artery bypass procedures grafting

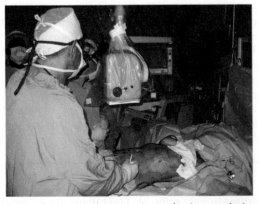

Fig. 1. Fluorescent laser angiography in use during perforator flap surgery. The camera is sterilely draped into the field to be directly manipulated by the operating surgeon.

procedures in 2005, and subsequently clearance for use during plastic and reconstructive and microsurgical procedures was received in 2007.

TECHNIQUE

Once the surgeon is ready to image, the camera is positioned and anesthesia gives a 5-mL bolus containing 2.5 mg ICG. No toxicity has been seen with total doses of 5 g/kg (400 mg in an 80-kg patient). Typical acquisition times are around 1 minute. If one is attempting to visualize and localize perforating blood vessels, the camera is turned on immediately to record the first blush. If perfusion is the goal, the camera is switched on 15 seconds after injection to maximize time for full tissue evaluation. As technology progresses these parameters may change, so one must check this with the particular vendor. If a second scan is desired, one should wait 5 minutes to allow washout of the ICG for optimal scanning. Some software development is under way to eliminate this wait by subtracting any background ICG still present. Current software, such as the SPY-Q (Novadaq/LifeCell) allows the data to be seen with colorimetric analysis for easier interpretation (**Fig. 2**). This software can analyze data and plot areas of maximal intensity, which correlates with best perfusion or perforator location.

APPLICATIONS
Documenting Tissue Perfusion/Angiosomes

By far the greatest utility of fluorescent angiography is the capability of visualizing perfusion in real time. Plastic surgeons require these vital data when evaluating tissues and creating flaps for reconstruction. The gold standard for evaluating perfusion is clinical judgment, and this judgment is acquired over a career. It is clinical judgment that allows seasoned surgeons to have lower rates of flap necrosis and healing problems, but it is difficult to teach this knowledge. It is a certain look and feel acquired through experience that allows the veteran to work within proper zones of perfusion we now call angiosomes.[26] It has been hypothesized that blood flow in a primary angiosome will support the tissue and support the secondary angiosome somewhat less, with any tertiary angiosomes being unreliable with a delay. With fluorescent angiography the hypothetical can now be directly visualized in real time by the surgeon and the information acted upon. As the ICG perfuses the tissues, the first blush corresponds with the primary angiosome. As this area begins to fade, the second angiosome lights up, somewhat fainter. No or little fluorescence is

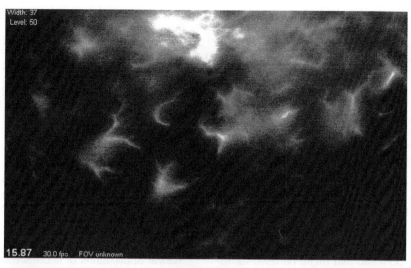

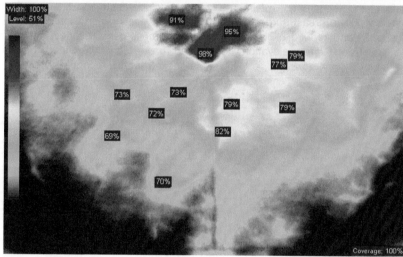

Fig. 2. Software is available for analyzing angiographic data and formatting it into easy-to-read color contour maps. These images are a summation of the angiogram and can be manipulated to look at peak fluorescence, maximum fluorescence, fastest fluorescence, and washout of fluorescence. Future software will be able to give valuable data on both arterial perfusion and venous egress.

seen in tertiary areas. While obvious via the infrared camera, clinically the differences are subtle at best (**Fig. 3**). Even the young surgeon without the benefit of experience can plan to use tissues only in the marked zones of good perfusion, thus lowering postoperative complications such as fat necrosis and wound-healing problems.

The information generated with fluorescent angiography can also be used to evaluate devitalized tissues in trauma and guide operative debridements. Devascularization that occurs with oncologic resections can also be evaluated before planning the reconstruction so that only the best perfused tissues are present in the wound. An example of this is the evaluation of mastectomy skin flaps in immediate reconstruction.[27] As

surgeons progress to nipple sparing and more frequent skin-sparing procedures, fluorescent angiography will be a vital guide to the safety of using such ischemic tissues (**Fig. 4**). Areas within mastectomy skin or nipples that do not fluoresce are ischemic, and reconstructive planning must account for this.

Another application of this technology is evaluation of local flaps created for reconstruction. These nonaxial or "random" flaps can have tenuous blood supply, and the decision to use them immediately or delay them needs to be made at the moment of creation. Fluorescent angiography provides the surgeon with additional data to make such a determination.[28,29] Examples include the inclusion of a perforator in the

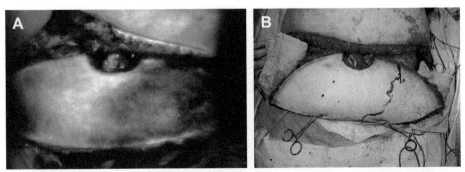

Fig. 3. Fluorescent angiogram of a transverse rectus abdominis myocutaneous (TRAM) flap (*A*) and clinical appearance of a TRAM flap (*B*). Subtle differences noted clinically are clearly noted on the angiogram. For the first time, angiographic zones can be directly observed in the elevated flaps, facilitating intraoperative decision making.

base of a random flap that might be used for re-surfacing a defect, and the creation of internal breast flaps for oncoplastic breast surgery. Both have nonaxial supply, and require clinical judgment of their perfusion after elevation for a successful result.

Newer applications of fluorescent angiography also include gastrointestinal and thoracic surgery, when evaluating perfusion of the bowel at critical anastomoses. In essence, any procedure that can have ischemia-related complications can benefit from this technology.

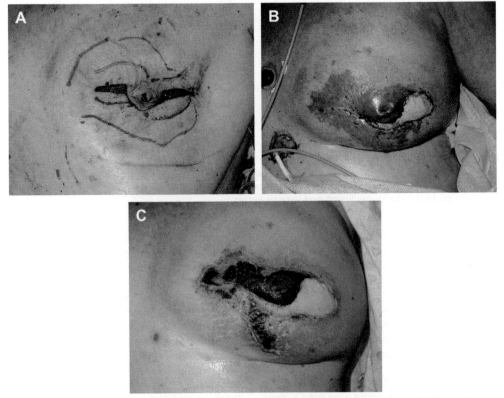

Fig. 4. Immediate reconstruction with deep inferior epigastric perforator (DIEP) flap and skin-sparing mastectomy. Outer line represents zone of no perfusion noted on fluorescent angiogram at 1 minute, inner line at 2 minutes. (*A*) Dark areas on angiogram were left and the DIEP skin was partially left to take any tension off the skin. Postoperative day 1. (*B*) Full-thickness loss of the nipple and surrounding skin at 2 weeks after operation. (*C*) The angiogram predicted the ultimate skin loss.

Decision Making in Perforator and Free-Flap Surgery

As we isolate a flap on a singular blood supply, we immediately reduce the amount of perfusion to that tissue. In primary zones this perfusion, though diminished, is adequate to nourish the transferred tissue.[30,31] With fluorescent angiography it is surprising to see how diminished the fluorescence is, even in well-executed flaps, when compared with surrounding tissues.[32] When we attempt to carry tissues on ever smaller vessels, we compromise circulation even more and increase the likelihood of ischemic complications such as fat necrosis and flap loss. As we raise these flaps and selectively clamp source vessels while performing fluorescent angiography, we can obtain valuable information on the actual zones of perfusion of each perforator and better assess the need for additional inflow to a flap. In pedicle flap surgery, this information may influence the decision to "supercharge" a flap with extra blood supply or "delay" the flap to give it extra time for the blood supply within the flap to reorganize.

Fluorescent angiography is often compared with computed tomographic angiography (CTA) for perforator localization. It must be borne in mind that fluorescent angiography is a superficial technology, giving information only on the most superficial 1 cm or so of any surface examined. In flaps of this thickness (arm, legs, scalp, thin abdomen), fluorescent angiography will compare favorably with CTA. It also has the advantage of being in real time, and perforators can be marked directly onto the tissues as visualized. CTA requires radiation exposure, a radiologist to read the study, and an element of error introduced as the surgeon translates the study information to the actual patient.[33] For thicker tissues greater than 1 cm, fluorescent angiography will be less accurate for perforator localization. The analogy with CTA is that whereas with CTA one is looking at the trunk and the roots of a tree, with fluorescent angiography one sees only the leaves of the tree. Decisions can still be made on first blush as to which tissues to include in flap design, but fascial location of the perforator is less certain as the distance to the fascia increases. Although the first blush of fluorescence is presumed to be the first and best perfused tissues, this has not been corroborated by clinical study. The same can be said of CTA: the largest noted perforator is presumed to have the best flow and distribution, but this has not been proved.

Postoperative Monitoring

Fluorescent angiography has a role in postoperative monitoring, but its utility at this point in time is limited by the availability of ICG dye and the fluorescent angiography machines in the recovery room or the postoperative ward. Some centers are using fluorescent angiography routinely for monitoring postoperative digit replants (R Buntic, MD, personal communication, 2009). These cases are particularly difficult to monitor postoperatively because other modalities like Doppler and temperature probes are unreliable. Other units place infrared cameras in endoscopes to evaluate hidden flaps in the aerodigestive space. As fluorescent angiography becomes more commonplace and the infrared cameras become more ubiquitous in our hospitals, the use of the technology for postoperative monitoring will increase.

Evaluation of the Microscopic Anastomoses

One of the early exciting uses of fluorescent angiography in plastic surgery was the evaluation of blood flow within arterial and venous conduits. Fluorescent angiography can be visually impressive and reassuring, as it shows blood entering then leaving a flap. One microscope manufacturer even incorporated the technology into its microscope just for this purpose. Over time, this application has become less relevant as clinical examination of flow with a strip test or implantable Doppler is preferred. However, there are cases of low flow in some flaps with a limited capillary bed (bone-only flaps, small muscle flaps) where flow is not always obvious and a Doppler signal is not obtainable, even though the tissues are viable. This drawback can be temporary, due to spasm, or may simply improve over time as the blood supply reorganizes within the tissue. Fluorescent angiography can immediately confirm inflow and egress to allay fears and document flow in the operating room, and eliminate the need to take down and evaluate an anastomosis, preventing the need for subsequent reanastomosis.

Documentation

In this day and age of protective medical documentation and malpractice liability, "if it is not documented in the record it did not happen." Fluorescent angiography can be helpful in certain cases where the physician appreciates the extra support of documentation of perfusion in tissues. Fluorescent angiography can be used to confirm or prove the existence of good perfusion during surgery or to document poor perfusion as the basis for intraoperative decision making. This documentation can also be used in support of insurance or legal claims. Images may also be used to educate family members or the patient on the procedure and to convey an idea of what things looked like during surgery or at the conclusion of the procedure.

FLUORESCENT ANGIOGRAPHY IN THE LITERATURE

In preclinical studies, infrared angiography with ICG has been used to assess the microcirculation of axial flaps,[28] predict necrosis in axial flaps,[34] visualize perforators for flap design,[35,36] and quantitate arterial and venous compromise based on ICG fluorescence intensity.[31] This preliminary animal work confirmed the usefulness of the technology and set the stage for clinical study.

Clinical studies of fluorescent angiography in reconstructive surgery have been numerous. Initial clinical studies focused on the utility of the technology in pedicled flaps.[29,37] This experience was extended to free-flap surgery. Studies have shown the utility of fluorescent angiography in flap design,[38] postoperative monitoring,[30,39] intraoperative anastomotic evaluation,[40,41] and intraoperative decision making.[1,42] Several studies have focused on breast reconstructive cases, including the mapping of pedicle transverse rectus abdominis myocutaneous (TRAM) flaps,[32] deep inferior epigastric perforator (DIEP) flaps,[43,44] and free superficial inferior epigastric artery (SIEA) flaps,[45] evaluation of mastectomy flaps,[44] and evaluation of flaps after inset,[44] all of which may influence intraoperative decision making. More clinical study certainly is warranted, and ultimately limits general acceptance and adoption of the technology in everyday use.

FUTURE DIRECTIONS

Fluorescent angiography is an attractive and easy-to-use technology that makes sense to plastic surgeons and reinforces their current concepts of blood supply and perfusion. We are only beginning to scratch the surface of the data being generated. As plastic surgeons, we would like to know how the level of fluorescence and the study in general can predict future necrosis or flap survival. With increasing experience and prospective study, it is hoped that this can be determined. If so, a software package that analyzes the data would be able to relate these likelihoods in an easy-to-understand numerical or visual format. In the future, those who are comfortable with CTA for locating perforators might benefit from integrated fluorescent angiography to help pick perforators by size, location, and perfusion (**Fig. 5**).

In addition, we clinically are often more concerned with venous egress as the source of necrosis or failure in our surgeries, but we continue

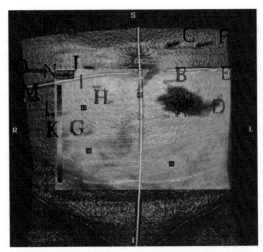

Fig. 5. CTA with fluorescent angiography overlay. This experimental work correlates preoperative perforator size and number estimates with a fluorescent angiography study performed at the time of surgery.

to focus on arterial inflow. Fluorescent angiography gives us the potential opportunity to evaluate venous egress by evaluating the disappearance of the ICG from the tissues. A clinical standard for inflow and outflow would be invaluable for intraoperative decision making.

Other idiosyncrasies of ICG also allow evaluation of the lymphatic and biliary systems, yet to be exploited in clinical care. One can certainly see the day when fluorescent angiography will be used in all aspects of a surgical case. In the case of breast reconstruction, this might include sentinel lymph node identification, mastectomy skin evaluation, perforator identification, flap dissection and preparation, and postoperative monitoring. Robots, endoscopes, and microscopes have already been outfitted with fluorescent angiographic technology, and it is only a matter of time before other equipment follows suit.[19]

SUMMARY

The old adage that states "there is no replacement for good clinical judgment" is as true today as ever. No amount of technology can replace surgical experience. However, this does not mean that technology cannot aid us in surgical decision making and in improving outcomes for our patients. Fluorescent angiography puts valuable information about blood flow in the hands of the operating surgeon in real time so that decisions can be made at the time of surgery to optimize outcomes.

Any fluorescent angiographic study is only a snapshot in time and because of this, its power to predict tissue survival will always have limits. Plastic surgeons know all too well that postoperative edema, dressings, blood pressure, nicotine use, patient activity, hematoma or seroma formation, infection, and countless other conditions can affect the ultimate outcome. But knowledge is power, and fluorescent angiography equips the operating surgeon with the added knowledge of perforator location, angiosome distribution, and tissue perfusion in the particular patient who is being operated on. If clinical experience is in part "reading the tea leaves," fluorescent angiography can help level the playing field for the less experienced and assist the experienced surgeon to navigate the anatomic variability inherent in all patients.

REFERENCES

1. Pestana IA, Coan B, Erdmann D, et al. Early experience with fluorescent angiography in free-tissue transfer reconstruction. Plast Reconstr Surg 2009; 123:1239–44.
2. Wood EH. Diagnostic applications of indicator-dilution technics in congenital heart disease. Circ Res 1962;10:531–68.
3. Samet P, Bernstein WH, Jacobs W, et al. Indicator-dilution curves in systemic arteriovenous fistulas. Am J Cardiol 1964;13:176–87.
4. Schillig S. Indicator-dilution techniques in the estimation of renal blood flow. Am Heart J 1964;68: 675–81.
5. Ketterer SG, Weigand BD. The excretion of indocyanine green and its use in the estimation of hepatic blood flow. Clin Res 1959;7:71.
6. Leevy CM, Stein SW, Cherrick GR, et al. Indocyanine green clearance: a test of liver excretory function. Clin Res 1959;7:290.
7. Flower RW, Hochhelmer BF. A clinical technique and apparatus for simultaneous angiography of the separate retinal and choroidal circulations. Invest Ophthalmol 1973;12:248–61.
8. Flower RW. Choroidal angiography using indocyanine green dye: a review and progress report. Opthalmol Dig 1974;36:18–27.
9. Ott P. Hepatic elimination of indocyanine green with special reference to distribution kinetics and the influence of plasma protein binding. Pharmacol Toxicol 1998;83(Suppl 2):1–48.
10. Desmettre T, Devoisselle JM, Mordon S. Fluorescence properties and metabolic features of indocyanine green (ICG) as related to angiography. Surv Ophthalmol 2000;45:15–27.
11. Benya R, Quintana J, Brundage B. Adverse reactions to indocyanine green: a case report and a review of the literature. Cathet Cardiovasc Diagn 1989;17:231–3.
12. Rubens FD, Ruel M, Fremes SE. A new and simplified method for coronary and graft imaging during CABG. Heart Surg Forum 2002;5:141–4.
13. Taggart DP, Choudhary B, Anastasiadis K, et al. Preliminary experience with a novel intraoperative fluorescence imaging technique to evaluate the patency of bypass grafts in total arterial revascularization. Ann Thorac Surg 2003;75:870–3.
14. Reuthebuch O, Kadner A, Lachat M, et al. Early bypass occlusion after deployment of nitinol connector devices. J Thorac Cardiovasc Surg 2004;127:1421–6.
15. Reuthebuch O, Häussler A, Genoni M, et al. Novadaq SPY: intraoperative quality assessment in off-pump coronary artery bypass grafting. Chest 2004;125: 418–24.
16. Balacumaraswami L, Abu-Omar Y, Anastasiadis K, et al. Does off-pump total arterial grafting increase the incidence of intraoperative graft failure? J Thorac Cardiovasc Surg 2004;128:238–44.
17. Takahashi M, Ishikawa T, Higashidani K, et al. SPY: an innovative intra-operative imaging system to evaluate graft patency during off-pump coronary artery bypass grafting. Interact Cardiovasc Thorac Surg 2004;3:479–83.
18. Balacumaraswami L, Abu-Omar Y, Choudhary B, et al. A comparison of transit-time flowmetry and intraoperative fluorescence imaging for assessing coronary artery bypass graft patency. J Thorac Cardiovasc Surg 2005;130:315–20.
19. Desai ND, Miwa S, Kodama D, et al. Improving the quality of coronary bypass surgery with intraoperative angiography: validation of a new technique. J Am Coll Cardiol 2005;46:1521–5.
20. Desai ND, Miwa S, Kodama D, et al. A randomized comparison of intraoperative indocyanine green angiography and transit-time flow measurement to detect technical errors in coronary bypass grafts. J Thorac Cardiovasc Surg 2006;132:585–94.
21. Desai ND, Moussa F, Singh SK, et al. Intraoperative fluorescence angiography to determine the extent of injury after penetrating cardiac trauma. J Thorac Cardiovasc Surg 2008;136:218–9.
22. Waseda K, Ako J, Hasegawa T, et al. Intraoperative fluorescence imaging system for on-site assessment of off-pump coronary artery bypass graft. JACC Cardiovasc Imaging 2009;2:604–12.
23. Sekijima M, Tojimbara T, Sato S, et al. An intraoperative fluorescent imaging system in organ transplantation. Transplant Proc 2004;36:2188–90.
24. Kubota K, Kita J, Shimoda M, et al. Intraoperative assessment of reconstructed vessels in living-donor liver transplantation, using a novel fluorescence imaging technique. J Hepatobiliary Pancreat Surg 2006;13:100–4.

25. Sanchez EQ, Chinnakotla S, Khan T, et al. Intraoperative imaging of pancreas transplant allografts using indocyanine green with laser fluorescence. Proc (Bayl Univ Med Cent) 2008;21:258–60.

26. Taylor GI, Gianoutsos MP, Morris SF. The neurovascular territories of the skin and muscles: anatomic study and clinical implications. Plast Reconstr Surg 1994;94:1–36.

27. Komorowska-Timek E, Gurtner GC. Intraoperative perfusion mapping with laser-assisted indocyanine green imaging can predict and prevent complications in immediate breast reconstruction. Plast Reconstr Surg 2010;125:1065–73.

28. Eren S, Rubben A, Krein R, et al. Assessment of microcirculation of an axial skin flap using indocyanine green fluorescence angiography. Plast Reconstr Surg 1995;96:1636–49.

29. Still H, Law E, Dawson J, et al. Evaluation of the circulation of reconstructive flaps using laser-induced fluorescence of indocyanine green. Ann Plast Surg 1999;42:266–74.

30. Holm C, Mayr M, Hofter E, et al. Intraoperative evaluation of skin-flap viability using laser-induced fluorescence of indocyanine green. Br J Plast Surg 2002;55:635–44.

31. Matsui A, Lee BT, Winer JH, et al. Real-time intraoperative near-infrared fluorescence angiography for perforator identification and flap design. Plast Reconstr Surg 2009;123:125e–7e.

32. Yamaguchi S, De Lorenzi F, Petit JY, et al. The perfusion map of the unipedicled TRAM flap to reduce postoperative partial necrosis. Ann Plast Surg 2004;53:205–9.

33. Rozen WM, Phillips TJ, Ashton MW, et al. Preoperative imaging for DIEA perforator flaps: a comparative study of computed tomographic angiography and Doppler ultrasound. Plast Reconstr Surg 2008;121:9–16.

34. Giunta RE, Holzbach T, Taskov C, et al. Prediction of flap necrosis with laser induced indocyanine green fluorescence in a rat model. Br J Plast Surg 2005;58:695–701.

35. Azuma R, Morimoto Y, Masumoto K, et al. Detection of skin perforators by indocyanine green fluorescence nearly infrared angiography. Plast Reconstr Surg 2008;122:1062–7.

36. Matsui A, Lee BT, Winer JH, et al. Image-guided perforator design using invisible near-infrared light and validation with x-ray angiography. Ann Plast Surg 2009;63:327–30.

37. Mothes H, Donicke T, Friedel R, et al. Indocyanine-green fluorescence video angiography used clinically to evaluate tissue perfusion in microsurgery. J Trauma 2004;57:1018–24.

38. Matsui A, Lee BT, Winer JH, et al. Quantitiative assessment of perfusion and vascular compromise in perforator flaps using a near-infrared fluorescence-guided imaging system. Plast Reconstr Surg 2009;124:451–60.

39. Holm C, Tegeler J, Mayr M, et al. Monitoring free flaps using laser-induced fluorescence of indocyanine green: a preliminary experience. Microsurgery 2002;22:278–87.

40. Holm C, Mayr M, Hofter E, et al. Assessment of the patency of microvascular anastomoses using microscope-integrated near-infrared angiography: a preliminary study. Microsurgery 2009;29:509–14.

41. Mohebali J, Gottlieb LJ, Agarwal JP. Further validation for use of the retrograde limb of the internal mammary vein in deep inferior epigastric perforator flap breast reconstruction using laser-assisted indocyanine green angiography. J Reconstr Microsurg 2010;26:131–5.

42. Krishnan KG, Schackert G, Steinmeier R. The role of near-infrared angiography in the assessment of post-operative venous congestion in random pattern, pedicled island and free flaps. Br J Plast Surg 2004;114:1361–2.

43. Lee BT, Matsui A, Hutteman M, et al. Intraoperative near-infrared fluorescence imaging in perforator flap reconstruction: current research and early clinical experience. J Reconstr Microsurg 2010;26(1):59–65.

44. Holm C, Mayr M, Hofter E, et al. Perfusion zones of the DIEP flap revisited: a clinical study. Plast Reconstr Surg 2006;117:37–43.

45. Holm C, Mayr M, Hofter E, et al. Interindividual variability of the SIEA Angiosome: effects on operative strategies in breast reconstruction. Plast Reconstr Surg 2008;122:1612–20.

Near-Infrared Spectroscopy in Autologous Breast Reconstruction

Amy S. Colwell, MD*, Randall O. Craft, MD

KEYWORDS

- Near-infrared spectroscopy • Autologous reconstruction
- Breast cancer • Free flap monitoring

Breast cancer is the most common cancer affecting women in North America, and a significant number of these women undergo mastectomy as part of their multidisciplinary treatment.[1] More than 80,000 postmastectomy breast reconstructions are performed in the United States each year, and this rate continues to increase annually.[2] Autologous tissue reconstruction reliably replicates both the appearance and feel of breast tissue while avoiding implantation of a foreign body. However, both free and pedicled flaps are subject to vaso-occlusive events that can lead to flap necrosis. Although the past decade has seen technical improvements in the execution of free tissue transfer, with success rates of 95% or higher,[3–5] total flap loss from microvascular failure is financially and emotionally stressful for both patient and surgeon. Because salvage rates are inversely proportional to the interval between the onset of vascular compromise and clinical recognition,[6] accurate and timely flap monitoring is critical.

The current benchmark for flap monitoring in autologous breast reconstruction is clinical observation of skin color, turgor, capillary refill, and dermal bleeding. However, more than 90% of surgeons use objective surveillance devices as an adjunct to clinical monitoring.[7] The qualities of an ideal monitoring device, as first described by Creech and Miller[8] in 1975, have remained unchanged. This device should be harmless to the patient and flap, rapidly responsive, accurate, reliable, and applicable to all types of flaps.[8,9] Despite the rapid progress in technology over the past 3 decades, no instrumentation has been introduced that satisfies all of these criteria. Temperature probes, implantable Dopplers, color duplex sonography, microdialysis, and laser Doppler flowmetry have all been described for monitoring free flaps with varying degrees of accuracy and cost-effectiveness. More recently, a new technology using near-infrared spectroscopy has emerged and shows promise as a clinically useful device for adjunctive monitoring in autologous breast reconstruction. This article focuses on the background, indications, and current clinical data for near-infrared spectroscopy.

BACKGROUND

Tissue viability depends on adequate oxygen delivery to meet cellular demands. Through evolution, a cardiovascular system developed in multicellular organisms to deliver this essential nutrient beyond the limits of simple diffusion. Because oxygen is poorly soluble in water and plasma, the respiratory pigment hemoglobin evolved to bind oxygen for transport and improve efficiency. Near-infrared spectroscopy uses the selective light absorption characteristics of hemoglobin to provide an assessment of perfusion and tissue oxygen saturation.

Financial Disclosures: Dr Colwell is a consultant for Allergan.
The Division of Plastic Surgery, Massachusetts General Hospital, 15 Parkman Street, WACC 435, Boston, MA 02114, USA
* Corresponding author.
E-mail address: acolwell@partners.org

Near-infrared spectroscopy measures scattering and absorption of calibrated wavelengths of near-infrared light, which is related to the oxygen content of the hemoglobin within the tissue monitored. Near-infrared light is able to penetrate skin, bone, and muscle to a depth of up to 20 mm with less scatter compared with light of shorter wavelengths. Near-infrared light is emitted from an optode into the tissue and then recovered by a receiving optode. Most frequently, these optodes are placed adjacent to one another with a single probe fixed to the area under investigation. The amount of light recovered from the tissue of interest depends on the intensity of incident light, degree of light scattering, and amount of chromophore absorption, and is subsequently continuously displayed real-time on an external monitor (**Figs. 1** and **2**).[10]

Chromophores selectively absorb light within tissue variably, depending on changes in oxygenation, resulting in a reduction of light intensity. The principal chromophores in biologic tissues are hemoglobin, myoglobin, and cytochrome c oxidase. In skin, the primary chromophore is hemoglobin, with a small contribution of chromophore by cytochrome c oxidase, and background absorption from other surrounding tissue. Because the degree of scattering can be assumed stable in the same tissue, and the intensity of emitted light is constant, changes in the recovered light can be attributed to the changes in the tissue concentrations of the chromophores.[10] Characteristic wavelengths of optical absorption for both oxygenated and deoxygenated hemoglobin enable both forms to be differentiated and the concentrations quantified.[11]

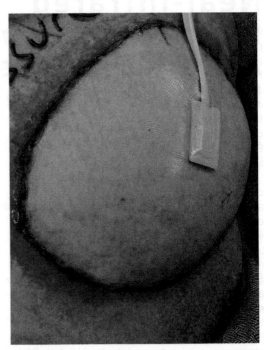

Fig. 2. Real-time noninvasive monitoring after autologous free flap reconstruction. In this patient, the probe is attached to the deep inferior epigastric artery perforator flap for postoperative monitoring.

Near-infrared spectroscopy instruments calculate the ratio of oxyhemoglobin and deoxyhemoglobin to generate a noninvasive real-time measurement of tissue oxygen saturation (StO_2). StO_2 is the percentage of hemoglobin bound to oxygen within the volume of tissue underneath the sensor patch. Any hemoglobin in the light path beneath the sensor, whether flowing in vascular space, pooled or extravascular, contributes to the StO_2. Changes in total tissue blood volume can also be calculated from the summation of concentrations of the oxygenated and deoxygenated hemoglobin, which may be useful in predicting venous insufficiency.[12–14]

CLINICAL APPLICATIONS

In 1977, Jobsis[11] was the first to note that biologic materials are relatively transparent in the near-infrared region of the spectrum, permitting photon transmission for monitoring cellular events, changes in tissue blood volume, and the average hemoglobin–oxyhemoglobin equilibrium. Mancini and colleagues[15] validated the functions of near-infrared spectroscopy in humans through measurements of skeletal muscle changes during forearm exercise.

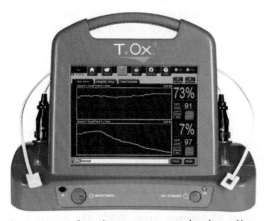

Fig. 1. Near-infrared spectroscopy technology. Near-infrared light is emitted from a central optic fiber and follows an elliptical path before it. The information is transferred to a console that provides continuous data monitoring.

To further determine the accuracy of near-infrared spectroscopy, Myers and colleagues[16] performed a comparison study between near-infrared spectroscopy (InSpectra Model 325, Hutchinson Technology, Hutchinson, MN, USA) and a carbon monoxide–oximeter in a closed circulating blood loop. They found a strongly positive correlation between the two measuring devices at oxygen saturation levels from 5% to 95%, confirming the validity of near-infrared spectroscopy.

Early clinical work with near-infrared spectroscopy was performed in trauma patients. McKinley and colleagues[17] showed the correlation of decreased oxygen saturation measurements with shock and subsequent organ dysfunction. Similarly, decreased near-infrared spectroscopy (InSpectra) measurements of muscle tissue oxygen saturation predicted poor perfusion, multi-organ dysfunction syndrome, and death after severe torso trauma.[18]

With this background of proven efficacy for detecting perfusion and oxygenation, the technology then naturally came under consideration for evaluating thrombo-occlusive events in plastic surgery. Irwin and colleagues[19] used near-infrared spectroscopy (Niro-500, Hamamatsu Photonics, United Kingdom) to measure StO_2 in the hind limb muscles of rabbits with arterial occlusion. They found a rapid decrease in oxygenation with occlusion of the common iliac artery and a rapid increase in oxygenation after restoration of flow.

In humans, Scheufler and colleagues[12] used the device in a pedicled transverse rectus abdominis musculocutaneous (TRAM) flap model. The authors analyzed 11 patients undergoing autologous breast reconstruction with an ipsilateral pedicled TRAM flap. Near-infrared spectroscopy (Multiscan OS10, NIOS-Medical Technologies, Germany) and color-coded duplex sonography measurements were obtained preoperatively, 1 day after surgery, and at late postoperative follow-up after 6 months. Zone IV was discarded in all reconstructions and not included in the measurements. Near-infrared spectroscopy was able to detect preoperative and postoperative differences of tissue hemoglobin content and oxygenation in the TRAM flap, and correlated with clinical examination and color-coded duplex sonography in detecting venous congestion in zone III. Because there was no partial or total flap loss in their series, they were not able to characterize critical thresholds for near-infrared spectroscopy in flaps with impaired perfusion that would result in subsequent necrosis.

The authors initially used near-infrared spectroscopy (ODISsey Tissue Oximeter, ViOptix, Inc, Fremont, CA, USA) to monitor free tissue transfer in an initial study of digit replantation in 48 patients and 64 digits.[20] At the time, serial quantitative fluoroscopy was considered the preferred objective monitor at the Buncke Clinic as an adjunct to clinical examination, but the monitoring was cumbersome and time-consuming, and therefore the authors sought alternative options. No significant differences in StO_2 measurements were seen between the digits that survived (61 digits) and the control digits. Three digit replantations failed. These failed digits had 30% to 70% lower StO_2 values than control digits. This finding correlated with serial quantitative fluoroscopy measurements. The authors concluded that near-infrared spectroscopy was able to accurately detect digit failure and that the technology may be valuable in monitoring digit replantation.

In a second series, the authors obtained intraoperative and postoperative tissue oxygen tension measurements with near-infrared spectroscopy in seven consecutive free flaps performed for breast reconstruction. Measurements were taken at baseline, after flap elevation, with clamping of inflow vessels, after vessel anastomosis, after flap insetting, and continuously during postoperative recovery.[21] Baseline tissue oxygen tissue measurements averaged 83% (range, 70%–99%), which is expected given the mixed oxygen saturation levels of capillary blood. When the vessels were clamped for flap transfer, StO_2 dropped an average of 33% (range, 25%–38%), but rapidly recovered to near preclamping values within 5 minutes after reanastomosis, and measurements remained stable for the next 48 hours (Fig. 3). Although no thromboembolic events occurred in this series, the intraoperative near-infrared spectroscopy measurements correlated with the iatrogenic surgical discontinuation of the blood supply, suggesting that near-infrared spectroscopy may be valuable for monitoring free flaps postoperatively.

Repez and colleagues[22] prospectively evaluated 50 free flaps used for autologous breast reconstruction in 48 patients by using continuous-wave near-infrared spectroscopy (InSpectra, Hutchinson Technology) for 72 hours of postoperative monitoring. In their study, 10 flaps (20%) developed 13 anastomosis thromboses (2 arterial and 11 venous). Near-infrared spectroscopy detected an abrupt decrease in StO_2 for arterial thromboses in all cases of flow failure before clinical evidence of vascular compromise, with no false-positives or false-negatives. Similarly, StO_2 levels dropped with venous occlusion, but the change was more gradual. The flap salvage rate was 70%, with an overall flap viability of 94%. The authors advocate

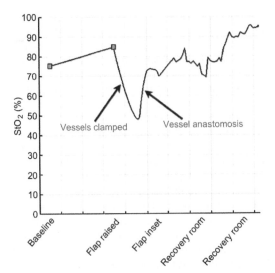

Fig. 3. Intraoperative and postoperative monitoring of free flaps with near-infrared spectroscopy. When the inflow vessels were clamped, StO_2 decreased significantly, but increased rapidly to preclamp values 5 to 10 minutes after reanastomosis. These values were maintained throughout the recovery period and on postoperative days 1 and 2. (*Reprinted from* Colwell AS, Wright L, Karanas Y. Near-infrared spectroscopy measures tissue oxygenation in free flaps for breast reconstruction. Plast Reconstr Surg 2008;121(5):344e–5e; with permission.)

near-infrared spectroscopy for monitoring flaps with a cutaneous component.

Keller[13] reviewed his initial experience with near-infrared spectroscopy (T.Ox Tissue Oximeter, ViOptix) in 30 patients undergoing autologous tissue perforator free flap breast reconstruction. In his series, the device detected two episodes of venous thrombosis before clinically apparent, which allowed for early flap salvage in both cases.

In a second larger series, Keller reported his outcomes in 208 autologous free flaps for breast reconstruction in 145 patients monitored with near-infrared spectroscopy intraoperatively and for 36 hours postoperatively.[14] Five patients had complications that were predicted by near-infrared spectroscopy before any clinical signs, allowing for expeditious flap salvage. The eight reoperations resulted from hematomas, venous congestion, and arterial thromboses. No flap losses occurred in the series. Based on his experience with these thromboembolic events, Keller devised a diagnostic algorithm for early prediction of vascular compromise based on an absolute StO_2 number and the StO_2 drop rate. In this study, a change in StO_2 of 20% or greater per hour predicted a vascular complication. In addition, an

absolute drop of StO_2 to less than 30% was also predictive of vascular compromise (**Figs. 4** and **5**).

Currently, the ViOptix T.Ox Tissue Oximeter and the Hutchinson InSpectra Oxygenation Monitor are the commercial near-infrared spectroscopy devices most widely reported for clinical use. The sensor patches are configured with photo detectors and laser light sources and transmit the data to a console with a display screen. A built-in mechanism determines signal strength that assists with sensor placement. Both systems allow for continuous, noninvasive monitoring with an ability to set high and low StO_2 alarms.

LIMITATIONS

Although promising, this emerging technology is not without limitations. The clinical usefulness of near-infrared spectroscopy measurement devices is in monitoring StO_2 over time rather than in isolated measurements. This concept is important for obtaining accurate, reliable information. Because the capillary density of skin is variable throughout the body, two spot measurements taken 1 or 2 cm apart may have different StO_2 values. Therefore, the clinical value for near-infrared spectroscopy depends on having a baseline measurement of a particular area and then observing changes in this value over time. Most clinical devices are used for continuous real-time monitoring, with the probe fixed to the skin in one spot. Therefore, false measurement changes can occur if the probe becomes detached with patient movement.

In addition, the diagnostic algorithm proposed by Keller is important for interpreting changes in StO_2. Small gradual changes (1%–10%) in measurements are normally observed as oxygen is weaned from the patient over the first 48 hours, and should not be misinterpreted as a vascular event as long as the StO_2 remains higher than 30% and is not rapidly dropping.

Other limitations of the technology result from devices being developed in different laboratories using proprietary algorithms without standardization across the industry. Therefore, the experience with and algorithms developed for one company's near-infrared spectroscopy device may not be transferrable to a device from another company. In addition, near-infrared spectroscopy light penetration may differ between systems according to variations in the selected wavelengths, technical and geometric factors, tissue characteristics, and chromophore concentrations.

Additionally, although near-infrared spectroscopy seems to be an accurate and sensitive tool for detecting vascular complications before overt

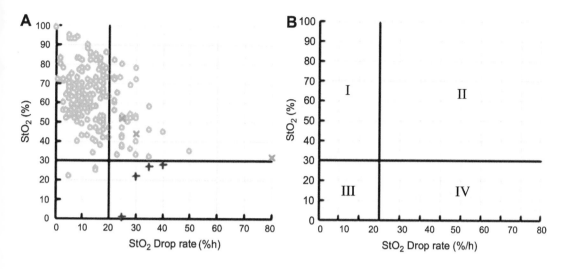

No complication

+ Complication

✖ Complication not fully developed upon intervention

Fig. 4. StO₂ and its drop rate can be combined to indicate possible hypoxia in a flap (*A*). All flaps with an absolute StO₂ of 30% or less and a change of StO₂ of 20% or greater per hour, sustained for more than 30 minutes, were those with complications (region IV in graph *B*). (*Reprinted from* Keller A. A new diagnostic algorithm for early prediction of vascular compromise in 208 microsurgical flaps using tissue oxygen saturation measurements. Ann Plast Surg 2009;62(5):538–43; with permission.)

clinical flap failure, the question remains whether the cost justifies its addition to standard clinical monitoring.

Proponents of near-infrared spectroscopy would argue that the cost of the system is offset by the need for less-intensive coverage by ancillary staff and residents performing hourly flap checks,

especially in the era of 80-hour work week mandates. With the proper setup, the console data can be accessed via the Internet, thus allowing surgeons to obtain information regarding viability of the flap while outside the hospital. With ballooning health care costs, a reliable monitoring device could actually provide a cost incentive for hospitals

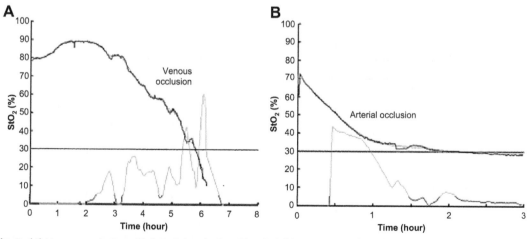

Fig. 5. (*A*) Venous occlusion. (*B*) Arterial occlusion. The dark blue curve on the top of each figure is directly from the StO₂ data, the red curve is the StO₂ average, and the blue curve in the bottom is the StO₂ drop rate. (*Reprinted from* Keller A. A new diagnostic algorithm for early prediction of vascular compromise in 208 microsurgical flaps using tissue oxygen saturation measurements. Ann Plast Surg 2009;62(5):538–43; with permission.)

if it allowed patients to avoid having to spend a night in the intensive care or postanesthesia care unit because hourly nursing checks were no longer needed.

The counterargument is that the success rate of free tissue transfer was reported to be 97% with clinical observation alone in a recent large series of 1140 consecutive flaps.[23] This high success rate with clinical observation sets a high standard for objective monitoring devices to improve on and suggests that selective use of devices in higher-risk cases could be more cost-effective.

The issues of standardization of technology and cost–benefit analysis are subjects for debate.

SUMMARY

Near-infrared spectroscopy has promise for providing a reliable means of continuous, noninvasive monitoring of flap oxygenation and perfusion. The series reviewed in this article have uniformly shown the ability of the technology to detect flap compromise. Although promising, the ultimate role of near-infrared spectroscopy within the monitoring algorithm of autologous breast reconstruction remains to be determined. The scope of near-infrared spectroscopy technology may reach other plastic surgery applications. Needs remain unmet in helping surgeons determine how much pedicled or free flap tissue will survive and in assessing the viability of the mastectomy skin envelope. Further research is needed to determine if near-infrared spectroscopy monitoring devices are suited for these and other applications.

REFERENCES

1. Nattinger AB. Variation in the choice of breast-conserving surgery or mastectomy: patient or physician decision making? J Clin Oncol 2005;23(24):5429–31.
2. Christian CK, Niland J, Edge SB, et al. A multi-institutional analysis of the socioeconomic determinants of breast reconstruction: a study of the National Comprehensive Cancer Network. Ann Surg 2006;243(2):241–9.
3. Smit JM, Acosta R, Zeebregts CJ, et al. Early reintervention of compromised free flaps improves success rate. Microsurgery 2007;27(7):612–6.
4. Jones NF, Jarrahy R, Song JI, et al. Postoperative medical complications–not microsurgical complications–negatively influence the morbidity, mortality, and true costs after microsurgical reconstruction for head and neck cancer. Plast Reconstr Surg 2007;119(7):2053–60.
5. Nakatsuka T, Harii K, Asato H, et al. Analytic review of 2372 free flap transfers for head and neck

6. Siemionow M, Arslan E. Ischemia/reperfusion injury: a review in relation to free tissue transfers. Microsurgery 2004;24(6):468–75.
7. Hirigoyen MB, Urken ML, Weinberg H. Free flap monitoring: a review of current practice. Microsurgery 1995;16(11):723–6 [discussion: 727].
8. Creech BJ, Miller SH. Evaluation of circulation in skin flaps. Boston: Little, Brown; 1975.
9. Smit JM, Zeebregts CJ, Acosta R, et al. Advancements in free flap monitoring in the last decade: a critical review. Plast Reconstr Surg 2010;125(1):177–85.
10. Scheufler O, Andresen R. Tissue oxygenation and perfusion in inferior pedicle reduction mammaplasty by near infrared reflection spectroscopy and color-coded duplex sonography. Plast Reconstr Surg 2003;111(3):1131–46.
11. Jobsis FF. Noninvasive, infrared monitoring of cerebral and myocardial oxygen sufficiency and circulatory parameters. Science 1977;198(4323):1264–7.
12. Scheufler O, Exner K, Andresen R. Investigation of TRAM flap oxygenation and perfusion by near infrared reflection spectroscopy and color-coded duplex sonography. Plast Reconstr Surg 2004;113(1):141–52 [discussion: 153–5].
13. Keller A. A new diagnostic algorithm for early prediction of vascular compromise in 208 microsurgical flaps using tissue oxygen saturation measurements. Ann Plast Surg 2009;62(5):538–43.
14. Keller A. Noninvasive tissue oximetry for flap monitoring: an initial study. J Reconstr Microsurg 2007;23(4):189–97.
15. Mancini DM, Bolinger L, Li H, et al. Validation of near infrared spectroscopy in humans. J Appl Physiol 1994;77:2740.
16. Myers DE, Anderson LD, Seifert RP, et al. Noninvasive method for measuring local hemoglobin oxygen saturation in tissue using wide gap second derivative near infrared spectroscopy. J Biomed Opt 2005;10:034017.
17. McKinley BA, Marvin RG, Cocanour CS, et al. Tissue hemoglobin O2 saturation during resuscitation of traumatic shock monitored using near infrared spectrometry. J Trauma 2002;48:637–42.
18. Cohn SM, Nathans AB, Moore FA, et al. Tissue oxygen saturation predicts the development of organ dysfunction during traumatic shock resuscitation. J Trauma 2007;62:44–55.
19. Irwin MS, Thorniley MS, Dore CJ, et al. Near infra-red spectroscopy: a non-invasive monitor of perfusion and oxygenation within the microcirculation of limbs and flaps. Br J Plast Surg 1995;48:14–22.
20. Colwell AS, Buntic RF, Brooks D, et al. Detection of perfusion disturbances in digit replantation using near infrared spectroscopy and serial quantitative fluoroscopy. J Hand Surg Am 2006;31(3):456–62.

reconstruction following cancer resection. J Reconstr Microsurg 2003;19(6):363–8 [discussion: 369].

21. Colwell AS, Wright L, Karanas Y. Near infrared spectroscopy measures tissue oxygenation in free flaps for breast reconstruction. Plast Reconstr Surg 2008;121(5):344e–5e.

22. Repez A, Oroszy D, Arnez ZM. Continuous postoperative monitoring of cutaneous free flaps using near infrared spectroscopy. J Plast Reconstr Aesthet Surg 2008;61(1):71–7.

23. Chubb D, Rozen WM, Whitaker IS, et al. The efficacy of clinical assessment in the postoperative monitoring of free flaps: a review of 1140 consecutive cases. Plast Reconstr Surg 2010;125(4):1157–66.

Use of the Implantable Doppler in Free Tissue Breast Reconstruction

Mazen I. Bedri, MD, Bernard W. Chang, MD*

KEYWORDS

- Free flap • Monitoring • Implantable Doppler
- Reconstruction

Free tissue transfer has advanced significantly as a reconstructive modality since its advent in the 1950s. Success rates have increased considerably as techniques have improved, with some investigators reporting less than 5% failure.[1–3] However, failure remains a very costly outcome in terms of time, resources, and patient morbidity, and delayed salvage efforts negatively affect the likelihood of flap success. Considerable attention is understandably directed to optimizing monitoring techniques and devices.

The growing list of indications and evolving techniques for free flaps have posed challenges to conventional monitoring techniques. Clinical examination can often fail to detect early thrombotic complications in free flaps. Hand-held Doppler ultrasonography and skin-surface temperature probes have limited uses in monitoring.[4] As a result, other monitoring methods have gained popularity more recently. Among these is the implantable Doppler system.

The implantable Doppler was first described by Swartz and colleagues[5] in 1988. The device allows for continuous invasive monitoring of blood flow through a vessel. This system uses an implantable 20-MHz pulsed ultrasonic probe to directly monitor the vascular anastomosis of a free flap.

TECHNIQUE

The electrode is typically mounted on a silicone cuff, which is wrapped gently but snugly around the venous pedicle (**Fig. 1**), and a thin wire connects the probe to the external monitor (**Fig. 2**).

The Doppler probe produces a pulsatile sound when attached to the artery and a venous hum when attached to the vein. The monitoring system is designed to be used for 5 to 10 days, after which the electrode is detached from the silicone cuff with minimal tension by pulling on the externalized wire.

INDICATIONS AND SETTINGS FOR THE IMPLANTABLE DOPPLER

The use of the implantable Doppler has been described by numerous investigators in a variety of settings, including reconstruction of the head and neck,[6–9] breast,[10–12] and extremities.[9,13] Guillemaud and colleagues[6] published one of the largest series on head and neck free flaps, mostly for oncologic defects, monitored via the implantable Doppler. In the retrospective series of 351 patients, the investigators found that a change in the Doppler signal increased the salvage rates from 61.5% to 92.0%, when compared with flaps in which no vascular complication was detected. The investigators attributed failures in detection to their choice of arterial monitoring.

A more recent retrospective review by Paydar and colleagues[7] of 169 consecutive free flaps for head and neck reconstruction also found a high overall salvage rate of 94.7%. Of the 19 flaps (4 buried flaps) that had changes in Doppler signals, the only flap failure occurred in 1 of the buried flaps. In contrast with Guillemaud and colleagues,[6] Paydar and colleagues[7] used the implantable Doppler to monitor venous flow, with

The authors have no financial interests to disclose.
Plastic and Reconstructive Surgery at Mercy Medical Center, 227 St Paul Place, Baltimore, MD 21202, USA
* Corresponding author.
E-mail address: bchang@mdmercy.com

Clin Plastic Surg 38 (2011) 309–312
doi:10.1016/j.cps.2011.03.016

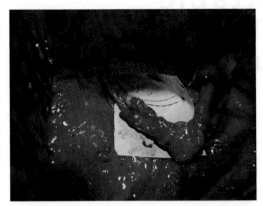

Fig. 1. The electrode is typically mounted on a silicone cuff, which is wrapped gently but snugly around the venous pedicle.

a sensitivity and specificity of 100% and 98.7%, respectively. None of the false-positive results required operative exploration after correlation with clinical examination, and there were no complications attributable to use of the implantable Doppler.

The implantable Doppler has also demonstrated applications in breast reconstruction. Rozen and colleagues[14] recently published their experience with 527 consecutive patients who underwent breast reconstruction using free tissue transfer, including deep inferior epigastric perforator, superficial inferior epigastric artery, and superior gluteal artery perforator. The investigators compared the efficacy of clinical monitoring in the first 426 patients with that of monitoring using the implantable Doppler in the subsequent 121 patients, with salvage rates of 66% and 80%, respectively. Although this difference was not significant, the investigators' meta-analysis of related literature showed a significant improvement in salvage rates associated with the use of this device. Smit and colleagues[11] similarly reviewed

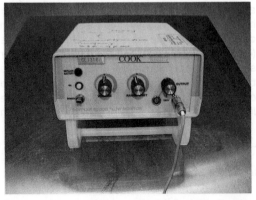

Fig. 2. A thin wire connects the implantable Doppler probe to the external monitor.

121 microvascular breast reconstructions retrospectively, all of which were monitored with implantable venous Doppler probes. A total of 14 flaps required salvage efforts, with an overall false-positive rate of 6.7% and a false-negative rate of 0%.

Whereas nonburied flaps can be monitored with a combination of clinical observation and implantable Doppler, buried flaps pose a particular challenge in postoperative care. In a retrospective review of 750 free flaps monitored only with conventional techniques, Disa and colleagues[4] reported that buried flaps had a significantly lower salvage rate of 0% compared with 77% for nonburied flaps. This result was associated with a significantly higher failure rate in buried flaps, 6.5% when compared with 1.8% in nonburied flaps. Unsurprisingly, the implantable Doppler has been used to monitor buried free flaps for head and neck, as well as for breast reconstruction.[6,7,10] Rozen and colleagues[10] published a unique series of 8 patients who underwent microvascular breast reconstruction using completely buried flaps; the investigators suggested that the implantable venous Doppler allows for the expanded use of such techniques.

RELIABILITY AND VALUE OF THE IMPLANTABLE DOPPLER

Advocates of the implantable Doppler point out that the monitoring technique is minimally invasive and adds little time or morbidity to free tissue transfers. Moreover, the device can detect flap compromise in settings in which other modalities are not easily implementable. However, these potential benefits are balanced against considerations of reliability and utility of the implantable Doppler in the setting of free flaps. In addition, the signal obtained from the device requires a learning curve for physicians as well as for hospital staff to interpret the analog sounds obtained. Lineaweaver[15] proposed a framework with which to evaluate the utility of any flap-monitoring device, based on the following 3 criteria: (1) the rate of false-positive results, (2) the device's sensitivity to true vascular complications, and (3) perhaps most importantly, the device's effect on the flap salvage rate.[15]

Sensitivity

Sensitivity of the implantable Doppler is critical in the timely management of flap compromise, and has improved since its advent in 1988. The device was originally described as a means of arterial monitoring.[5] Swartz and colleagues[16] noted a marked improvement in sensitivity, from 66.7%

to 100%, when monitoring the venous pedicle rather than the artery.[16] In a relatively recent retrospective series, the investigators relied on arterial Doppler monitoring in an effort to decrease the rate of false-positive signal changes; the study documented a sensitivity of only 65.8%.[6] However, the overwhelming majority of studies over the past decade pertain to venous Doppler monitoring, with a sensitivity of 100% being frequently reported.[7,9,11,17–19]

Specificity

In contrast, the specificity of the implantable Doppler has generated greater debate regarding its reliability as a monitoring technique. Studies quote a wide range of false-positive rates for the implantable Doppler, as high as 88%.[8,12,19] The clinical implication of such a poor positive predictive value is an unacceptable number of needless operative explorations.[19] Some investigators submit that adjunct monitoring techniques, such as eternalizing a segment of the buried flap[8] or the using confirmatory tests such as color duplex sonography,[19] are useful in averting unnecessary trips back to the operating theater.

Flap Salvage Rate

Ultimately, the utility of the implantable Doppler is measured by any attributable improvement in outcomes. There are studies suggesting that the implantable Doppler does not yield any true difference in salvage rates.[12] In contrast, other studies report relatively high salvage rates for buried and nonburied flaps monitored by the device.[7,9] Some data demonstrate trends toward improved salvage rates, or even statistical significance, associated with the implantable Doppler when compared with clinical monitoring.[13,14,20] One large retrospective study showed significantly improved flap success rates with the implantable Doppler but only within specific subspecialties including ear, nose, throat; breast reconstruction; and orthopedic oncology.[20] Such differences suggest that the device may contribute to the management of free flaps in varying degrees, depending on the nature of reconstruction.

SUMMARY

The implantable Doppler is advocated as an effective modality for detecting flap compromise. However, false-positive signal changes are not without cost and can only be mitigated with good surgical technique, clinical judgment, and the possible use of other imaging techniques. In addition, the data from numerous retrospective studies remain seemingly inconclusive as to whether the device ultimately improves outcomes in free tissue transfers.

Given the low rate of flap complications in most series, a much larger total sample size may be needed to unmask differences in salvage rates between the implantable Doppler and conventional methods of monitoring. Further, the true value of the implantable Doppler may be rooted in its ability to monitor flaps in which other modalities are not practicable. It may even afford surgeons the confidence to expand their microvascular techniques.

REFERENCES

1. Schusterman MA, Miller MJ, Reece GP, et al. A single center's experience with 308 free flaps for repair of head and neck cancer defects. Plast Reconstr Surg 1994;93(3):472–8 [discussion: 479–80].
2. Kroll SS, Schusterman MA, Reece GP, et al. Choice of flap and incidence of free flap success. Plast Reconstr Surg 1996;98(3):459–63.
3. Hidalgo DA, Disa JJ, Cordeiro PG, et al. A review of 716 consecutive free flaps for oncologic surgical defects: refinement in donor-site selection and technique. Plast Reconstr Surg 1998;102(3):722–32 [discussion: 733–4].
4. Disa JJ, Cordeiro PG, Hidalgo DA. Efficacy of conventional monitoring techniques in free tissue transfer: an 11-year experience in 750 consecutive cases. Plast Reconstr Surg 1999;104(1):97–101.
5. Swartz WM, Jones NF, Cherup L, et al. Direct monitoring of microvascular anastomoses with the 20-MHz ultrasonic Doppler probe: an experimental and clinical study. Plast Reconstr Surg 1988;81(2):149–61.
6. Guillemaud JP, Seikaly H, Cote D, et al. The implantable Cook-Swartz Doppler probe for postoperative monitoring in head and neck free flap reconstruction. Arch Otolaryngol Head Neck Surg 2008;134(7):729–34.
7. Paydar KZ, Hansen SL, Chang DS, et al. Implantable venous Doppler monitoring in head and neck free flap reconstruction increases the salvage rate. Plast Reconstr Surg 2010;125(4):1129–34.
8. Ferguson RE Jr, Yu P. Techniques of monitoring buried fasciocutaneous free flaps. Plast Reconstr Surg 2009;123(2):525–32.
9. Kind GM, Buntic RF, Buncke GM, et al. The effect of an implantable Doppler probe on the salvage of microvascular tissue transplants. Plast Reconstr Surg 1998;101(5):1268–73 [discussion: 1274–5].
10. Rozen WM, Whitaker IS, Wagstaff MJ, et al. Buried free flaps for breast reconstruction: a new technique using the Cook-Swartz implantable Doppler probe for postoperative monitoring. Plast Reconstr Surg 2010;125(4):171e–2e.

11. Smit JM, Whitaker IS, Liss AG, et al. Post operative monitoring of microvascular breast reconstructions using the implantable Cook-Swartz Doppler system: a study of 145 probes & technical discussion. J Plast Reconstr Aesthet Surg 2009;62(10):1286–92.

12. Whitaker IS, Rozen WM, Chubb D, et al. Postoperative monitoring of free flaps in autologous breast reconstruction: a multicenter comparison of 398 flaps using clinical monitoring, microdialysis, and the implantable Doppler probe. J Reconstr Microsurg 2010;26(6):409–16.

13. Rozen WM, Enajat M, Whitaker IS, et al. Postoperative monitoring of lower limb free flaps with the Cook-Swartz implantable Doppler probe: a clinical trial. Microsurgery 2010;30(5):354–60.

14. Rozen WM, Chubb D, Whitaker IS, et al. The efficacy of postoperative monitoring: a single surgeon comparison of clinical monitoring and the implantable Doppler probe in 547 consecutive free flaps. Microsurgery 2010;30(2):105–10.

15. Lineaweaver W. Techniques of monitoring buried fasciocutaneous free flaps. Plast Reconstr Surg 2009;124(5):1729–31.

16. Swartz WM, Izquierdo R, Miller MJ. Implantable venous Doppler microvascular monitoring: laboratory investigation and clinical results. Plast Reconstr Surg 1994;93(1):152–63.

17. Oliver DW, Whitaker IS, Giele H, et al. The Cook-Swartz venous Doppler probe for the post-operative monitoring of free tissue transfers in the United Kingdom: a preliminary report. Br J Plast Surg 2005; 58(3):366–70.

18. Pryor SG, Moore EJ, Kasperbauer JL. Implantable Doppler flow system: experience with 24 microvascular free-flap operations. Otolaryngol Head Neck Surg 2006;135(5):714–8.

19. Rosenberg JJ, Fornage BD, Chevray PM. Monitoring buried free flaps: limitations of the implantable Doppler and use of color duplex sonography as a confirmatory test. Plast Reconstr Surg 2006; 118(1):109–13 [discussion: 114–5].

20. Schmulder A, Gur E, Zaretski A. Eight-year experience of the Cook-Swartz Doppler in free-flap operations: microsurgical and reexploration results with regard to a wide spectrum of surgeries. Microsurgery 2011;31(1):1–6.

Noninvasive Tissue Oximetry

Alex Keller, MD[a,b],*

KEYWORDS

- Noninvasive flap monitoring • Near infrared spectroscopy
- Monitoring • Free flap monitoring • Breast reconstruction
- Microvascular surgery • DIEP flap • Thrombosis

Noninvasive tissue oximetry has proven to be an extremely valuable tool to assist in the surgical decision-making process during various stages of autologous tissue breast reconstruction, in both the intraoperative and postoperative setting. Tissue oximetry is a sensitive measure of real-time changes in local tissue oxygen saturation (StO_2). It is useful for intraoperative assessment of flap physiology, perforator selection, mapping to assist in the selection of tissue with the best chance of survival, and in identifying circulatory compromise during postoperative flap monitoring.[1–3]

Although any monitoring technique serves as an adjunct to clinical evaluation, improvements in monitoring technologies can provide information in many cases that identify a problem before it becomes obvious on clinical evaluation.[1,2] Flap salvage is inversely proportional to the time interval between the onset of ischemia and its clinical recognition.[4] With this in mind, and with the availability of objective data from newer flap assessment technologies, monitoring and evaluation of a flap with information other than clinical observation has become even more relevant in optimizing outcomes in autologous breast reconstruction. Successful monitoring should provide rapid detection of vascular problems and be simple to use.[5]

Autologous breast flap monitoring techniques currently employed include laser Doppler flowmetry, internal and external thermometry, internal and external Doppler monitoring, pulse oximetry, transcutaneous oxygen monitoring, quantitative fluorescein fluorescence, fluorescent angiography, and near infrared spectroscopy (NIRS). The most useful monitoring technique would be noninvasive, sensitive, accurate, quantitative, and provide continuous information. Techniques that are currently the most popular include the external Doppler, the implantable Doppler, and near infrared spectroscopy. The external Doppler technique is limited in its ability to reliably access the recipient vessels. The implantable Doppler technique has the ability to evaluate flow in both the arterial and venous system.[6,7] Partial occlusions require clinical interpretation of the Doppler sounds.[7] Additionally, accidental dislodgement of the probe leads to loss of signal. Fluorescent angiography is a new technique that provides reliable information regarding flow into the flap but provides only a snapshot in time consistent with the injection of a dye.[8] The equipment is bulky and is neither designed for nor practical for postoperative flap monitoring.

Tissue oximetry using near infrared spectroscopy is a noninvasive technique for flap monitoring and evaluation. The technique readily lends itself to continuous monitoring of the tissue.[1,2,9] Because of the easy placement of the sensor, different areas of the flap can be evaluated intraoperatively in real time during flap elevation and transfer. In addition, noninvasive near infrared tissue oximetry can be used to evaluate the viability of mastectomy skin flaps and assist in surgical decision making. Clinically, in many

Disclosure: The author is a medical consultant and holds stock options in ViOptix, Inc.
[a] Division of Plastic Surgery, Department of Surgery, North Shore Long Island Jewish Health System, 270-05 76th Avenue, New Hyde Park, NY 11040, USA
[b] Division of Plastic Surgery, Department of Surgery, New York University Medical Center, 550 First Avenue, New York, NY 10016, USA
* 900 Northern Boulevard, Great Neck, NY 11021.
E-mail address: Akplastic@gmail.com

Clin Plastic Surg 38 (2011) 313–324
doi:10.1016/j.cps.2011.03.017

situations, such as in deeply pigmented skin or bruised mastectomy flaps, the evaluation of the mastectomy skin flap has proven to be a difficult clinical decision.

How does one come to trust and rely on a new monitoring device? First, there is the recognition that such a device would be useful. This recognition is basically an acknowledgment of our human limitations. Next, one must have some understanding of how the technology works and what the information represents. Normal physiology of a revascularized flap and abnormal physiology must be recognized. Lastly, when a level of confidence is gained, additional uses of the device can be applied to help evaluate the health and potential viability of a flap or piece of tissue.

Motivation for use of a continuous monitoring device after free flap transfer can be for a variety of reasons. Well-educated paraprofessionals, especially in the private-practice arena, are often relied upon to evaluate the viability of a flap. In a university setting it is most often the resident's responsibility for flap evaluation. With overworked staff and reduced numbers of staff, the need for adjunctive monitoring is apparent.

Khouri[10] reported in 1992 that the single most important factor in determining success of free tissue transfer was the experience of the surgeon. He reported a thrombosis rate of 3.7% with a 66% salvage rate for timely operative revisions. He also noted that most surgeons of that era relied on clinical observation alone as their method of monitoring a flap. Three years later, Hirigoyen[11] reported from a questionnaire sent to 211 microsurgery centers that in 90% of cases adjunctive monitoring devices were used and that only 10% of surgeons rely solely on clinical evaluation for flap monitoring.

In 2010 Smit and colleagues[12] conducted a literature review of flap monitoring methods over the last decade. They concluded that although clinical monitoring of a flap is inexpensive, their results do not favor this as the sole method of flap monitoring because of the longer response time to diagnose vascular compromise. In comparing near infrared spectroscopy, the implantable Doppler, and laser Doppler flowmetry, they concluded that near infrared spectroscopy has the greatest potential in becoming the ideal monitoring method. They reported that flap monitoring with near infrared spectroscopy was reliable and had 100% positive and negative predictive values.

Although the success rate for free flap transfer in the hands of most experienced microsurgeons is 95% or better,[12] there is a take-back rate for vascular compromise in 6% to 25% of cases.[5,13] Successful salvage of these take backs is much dependent upon the time interval from the onset of the event to its correction. Therefore, earlier recognition of vascular compromise is paramount for an ultimately high success rate in free tissue transplantation.

Near infrared spectroscopy for monitoring of autologous breast reconstructions has been studied in the author's practice using the ViOptix T.Ox Tissue Oximeter (**Fig. 1**) manufactured by ViOptix, Inc (Fremont, CA, USA) in 505 consecutive free flap breast reconstructions. Flaps used were either abdominal flaps (deep inferior epigastric

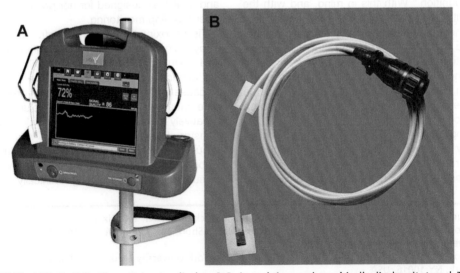

Fig. 1. (*A*) The ViOptix T. Ox Tissue Oximeter displays StO$_2$ in real time and graphically displays its trend. There are alarms for the StO$_2$ and rate of drop of StO$_2$. (*B*) The monitor cable is connected to a sensor that attaches to the tissue to be monitored with the supplied adhesive pad. The sensor is 1 cm in size and has 2 emitters and 4 light detectors. (*Courtesy of* ViOptix Inc, Fremont, CA; with permission.)

perforator [DIEP] or superficial inferior epigastric perforator [SIEP]) or gluteal flaps (superficial gluteal artery perforator [s-GAP]). Monitoring began in the operating room and continued for a period of 36 hours postoperatively. The study group consisted of 305 patients with 135 single breast reconstructions, 170 bilateral breast reconstructions, and 30 patients who had 2 flaps used to make a single larger breast. Results of some of these reconstructions have been published in 2 previous articles.[1,14] The ViOptix T.Ox Tissue Oximeter has been improved multiple times over the last 5 years. The current model being used includes a calculation, display, and alarm for the rate of drop of the tissue oxygen saturation, has dual channels to monitor 2 flaps simultaneously, and incorporates Wi-Fi. Wi-Fi allows the surgeon to check on the flap remotely using any device that has an Internet connection and browser. This feature allows the surgeon to interpret a trend without having to rely on a report from an observer in the hospital.

HOW TISSUE OXIMETRY WORKS

Tissue oximetry uses near infrared spectroscopy to measure the tissue oxygen saturation (StO_2). In the near infrared spectrum, we are only interested in those compounds whose absorption properties are oxygen dependent. The main compounds in the body whose near infrared absorption properties are oxygen dependent are hemoglobin, myoglobin, and the cytochromes. By limiting observations to changes in absorption, background contributions from the tissue can be eliminated.[15] The T.Ox Tissue Oximeter uses optical tissue characterization of light scattering and absorption in the near infrared spectrum, which is related to the oxygen content of the hemoglobin in that particular tissue. The light scattering occurs in tissue and characterizes that tissue's optical properties. It is the chromophores in the tissue that are responsible for the absorption of light. Water and hemoglobin are the major absorbers responsible for these changes in the near infrared spectrum. The calculation of tissue oxygen saturation is based upon this absorption and scattering.[16] The depth of measurement depends on the distance between the emitters and the sensors. The ViOptix T.Ox measures StO_2 at a depth up to 10 mm. The ViOptix T.Ox sensor has 2 emitters and 4 detectors of NIR light. StO_2 numbers displayed on the monitor are an average of multiple values.

NORMAL PHYSIOLOGY

Tissue oxygen saturation values are not the same as the oxygen saturation readings from a pulse oximeter. StO_2 is a local measure of how well a given piece of tissue is oxygenated. Oxygen saturation (SO_2) from either an arterial blood gas or a pulse oximeter is a systemic measure of how well the blood is oxygenated. There is more variation within a range of normals with tissue oxygen saturation. Tissue oxygen saturation values can vary considerably from patient to patient for the same location because of patients' unique physiologic profiles or comorbidities. To determine the health of a flap and evaluate if perfusion has been compromised by the flap harvest and transfer, tissue oxygen saturation readings should be taken before beginning the surgery. These readings are the baseline values for that flap for that particular patient. The StO_2 loosely correlates with flap perfusion and indirectly with perforator size. After the flap has been transferred one would not expect the tissue oxygen saturation readings to be significantly higher than the preoperative baseline level. Additionally, the converse of that is also true for a well-perfused flap.

When patients are receiving supplemental oxygen, tissue oxygen saturation increases (**Fig. 2**). When patients change position, tissue oxygen saturation can also change (**Fig. 3**). Just before patients are extubated, the anesthesiologist places patients on 100% oxygen, which increases tissue oxygen saturation. If patients are extubated in the operating room and then transported to the postanesthesia care unit, one would expect the StO_2 of the flap to decrease (**Fig. 4**). Conditions that can cause the SO_2 to drop, such as pneumothorax, pulmonary embolism, or an arrhythmia, can also cause a decrease in the StO_2.

ABNORMAL PHYSIOLOGY

With an understanding that near infrared spectroscopy measures the ongoing changing tissue oxygen saturation and therefore flap perfusion, we are now equipped to examine the abnormal events that we would like to capture. These events include both complete and incomplete arterial or venous compromise. Total arterial occlusion can be thought of as an event where the tissue or flap continues to metabolize and hence consume oxygen in a warm environment without the supply being replenished. (ie, warm ischemia). Initially, in evaluating the ViOptix T.Ox a lower limit of tissue oxygen saturation of 30% was used as the critical value below which a flap would not survive. Back testing this data revealed that the rate of drop of the StO_2 could be used as an earlier predictor of flap ischemia. A rate of decay/time $(\Delta StO_2)/(\Delta t)$ of 20% or greater when sustained for 30 minutes or more predicted vascular compromise (**Fig. 5**).[1]

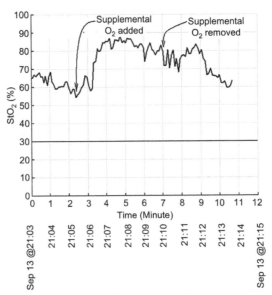

Fig. 2. A tissue oximetry sensor is placed on the patient's thumb and the patient is breathing room air. SO_2 on the pulse oximeter is 97%. Supplemental O_2 with a 40% face tent was added. SO_2 rose to 99%. Supplemental O_2 was removed and StO_2 declined.

With venous occlusion, either partial or complete, blood does not freely exit the tissue. Again there is a drop in tissue oxygen saturation that can be readily detected. Venous insufficiency can be predicted by changes in total blood volume, which is calculated from the summation of the concentrations of oxygenated and deoxygenated hemoglobin.[2] Clinically, one sees the

flap becoming boggy and tense with the development of ecchymosis. The clinical findings lag behind the drop in StO_2. Pure venous occlusion was created in a DIEP flap that was not elevated or needed (**Fig. 6A**).

With arterial occlusion, blood does not enter the tissue and as the flap continues to metabolize, StO_2 will fall. Pure arterial occlusion was created

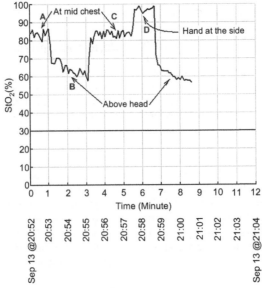

Fig. 3. A tissue oximetry sensor is placed on the patient's thumb and the SO_2 is 97% on room air. The graph before point A is with the patient's hand at midchest level. At point A the hand is raised to above the patient's head and at point B again to midchest level. At point C the patient's hand is allowed to hang at the side and at point D the hand is again raised to above the head.

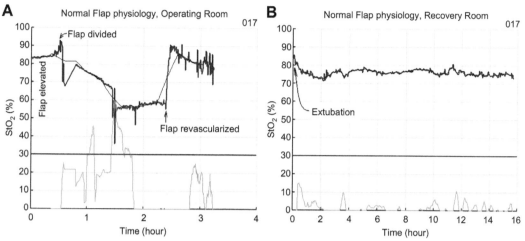

Fig. 4. Normal flap physiology when the flap is in (*A*) the operating room and (*B*) the recovery room. Note: the dark blue curve on the top of each figure corresponds to the StO$_2$ measurement data, the red curve corresponds to the running average of the StO$_2$, and the blue curve in the bottom represents the StO$_2$ drop rate (in StO$_2$% units per hour). (*From* Keller A. A new diagnostic algorithm for early prediction of vascular compromise in 208 microsurgical flaps using tissue oxygen saturation measurements. Ann Plast Surg 2009;62(5):540; with permission.)

in a DIEP flap that was neither elevated nor needed (see **Fig. 6B**). Clinically this can be difficult to identify in a pale flap. In patients with poor perfusion, for reasons such as hypotension or a low hematocrit, capillary refill can be hard or impossible to see. In such cases even pin pricks of the flap can produce results that are difficult to evaluate. A constant value on the tissue oximeter without

a drop in StO$_2$ should give the clinician confidence to investigate and correct these problems before concluding that reoperation for anastomotic exploration is necessary.

There is controversy as to whether near infrared spectroscopy can determine the difference between arterial or venous thrombosis and identify partial vascular compromise.[17] Repez and colleagues[2]

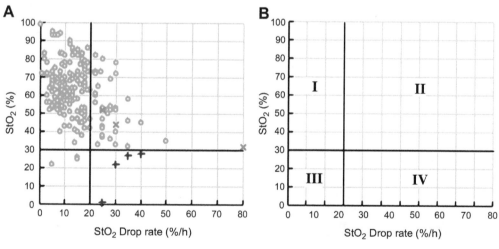

○ No complication

✚ Complication

✖ Complication not fully developed
   upon intervention

Fig. 5. (*A*) StO$_2$ and its drop rate can be combined to indicate possible hypoxia in a flap. All flaps with StO$_2$ less than or equal to 30% and Δ StO$_2$/Δ t greater than or equal to 20% per hour sustained for more than 30 minutes were flaps with complications (region IV in [*B*]). (*From* Keller A. A new diagnostic algorithm for early prediction of vascular compromise in 208 microsurgical flaps using tissue oxygen saturation measurements. Ann Plast Surg 2009;62(5):541; with permission.)

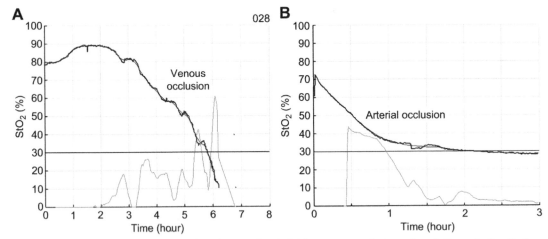

Fig. 6. (*A*) Venous occlusion. (*B*) Arterial occlusion. The dark blue curve on the top of each figure is directly from the StO$_2$ data, the red curve for the StO$_2$ average, and the blue curve in the bottom for the StO$_2$ drop rate. (*From* Keller A. A new diagnostic algorithm for early prediction of vascular compromise in 208 microsurgical flaps using tissue oxygen saturation measurements. Ann Plast Surg 2009;62(5):543; with permission.)

distinguished between arterial and venous thrombosis by analyzing levels of tissue hemoglobin. With arterial thrombosis, levels of tissue hemoglobin fell and with venous thrombosis levels of tissue hemoglobin rose. Of note is that the tissue hemoglobin changes occur late compared with the steep decline in the StO$_2$ that occurs with the thrombotic event.

Normal variations in tissue oxygen saturation never sustain a drop rate of greater than 20% for more than 30 minutes. That is not to say that these drops in tissue oxygen saturation are not a cause for concern. With experience, one comes to realize that they represent normal physiologic variations.

The flap in **Fig. 7** represents an abrupt drop in StO$_2$. In addition, the flap took on a mottled, but not blue, appearance. It is hypothesized that the event may have been caused by a small embolus.

Observing the flap expectantly, tissue oxygen saturation improved.

Knowing how a flap responds physiologically is useful in flap evaluation. In patients who are upright and sitting in a chair, the flap StO$_2$ will routinely drop. Patients are told that if the StO$_2$ numbers drop more than 10 to 15 points, they should go back to bed and lie flat. In a healthy flap, the StO$_2$ will increase.

Low flow (2 L/min) nasal oxygen is used for all patients when they are near the oxygen source, which increases flap StO$_2$ and gives a small extra margin of time in the event of flap ischemia. Additionally, adding supplemental oxygen or increasing its concentration should cause the StO$_2$ to increase. If it does not, one should be highly suspicious that the flap is vascularly compromised. The addition

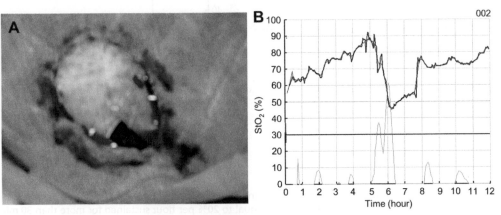

Fig. 7. (*A*) The flap island. (*B*) The StO$_2$ changes measured during the event. (*From* Keller A. A new diagnostic algorithm for early prediction of vascular compromise in 208 microsurgical flaps using tissue oxygen saturation measurements. Ann Plast Surg 2009;62(5):542; with permission.)

or increase in concentration of supplemental O_2 is a simple, easy test to use in the armamentarium of flap evaluation.

FLAP MONITORING

Flap monitoring begins in the operating room where baseline readings are taken in the medial and lateral portions of the flap just before the surgical procedure is begun. Although additional readings may be taken during the flap elevation in cases of a long flap crossing the midline, viability of tissue across a scar, or the need for an additional perforator, routinely, readings are not taken again until just before flap transfer. At this point, readings are obtained at the medial and lateral portions of the flap to confirm that flap perfusion has not changed from the presurgical levels. Once the flap is transferred, the tissue oxygenation sensor is applied to the area of skin that will be exposed when the flap is inset and the perfusion is monitored. While the operation continues (ie, a second flap being raised, abdominal closure), the graphical display on the tissue oxygenation monitor screen and StO_2 percentages displayed are constantly reviewed. The flap has been ischemic during the transfer and one looks for a rebound in the StO_2. A hyperemic response with an overshooting of the baseline StO_2 is expected. Another explanation for the slight rise in StO_2 was offered by Najefi.[18] His group thinks that the rise in StO_2 is caused by autonomic denervation of the flap cutaneous vessels during dissection and an inflammatory reaction at the wound margin.[18] In either case, failure to see this rise is a cause for concern.

In the gluteal flap represented in **Fig. 8**, analysis of the StO_2 tracing fails to show any elevation in the StO_2 after flap revascularization. This finding was an early indicator of arterial thrombosis. Although the flap bled on pinprick, in retrospect it bled poorly. When the pedicle was finally reexamined, there was an arterial thrombosis.

The StO_2 sensor is removed from the flap during insetting because the intensity and frequency of the operating room light interferes with StO_2 readings. Additionally, the sensor cable is in the way during this portion of the procedure.

At the conclusion of the flap insetting a spot is chosen on the flap for continuous postoperative monitoring. After sampling different areas of the flap, only one spot is chosen for monitoring. The spot is selected based on observations of good signal quality displayed on the T.Ox monitor and is representative of multiple sampled areas. A spot with abnormally high StO_2 is to be avoided. If the sensor is placed directly over a small vessel the oxygen saturation of the blood in that vessel is being measured. This measurement is not representative of perfusion or tissue oxygen saturation of the flap. For instance, an StO_2 of 99% would not be expected in tissue but might be expected in an artery. If the sensor is placed directly over an artery, SO_2 rather than StO_2 is being measured. The data displayed would not provide the clinician with timely information in the event of a vascular compromise. The rate of fall of the oxygen saturation in a vessel would be less than the rate of fall in tissue that is metabolizing. The slower rate of fall of oxygen saturation in a vessel as compared to tissue that was metabolizing would cause an unnecessary delay in being alerted to vascular compromise of the flap. Having taken the precautions previously described to have a uniformly healthy flap, the assumption is now made that this single point is representative of the entire flap.

Because there are variations in the StO_2 in different areas of the flap, care is taken to secure

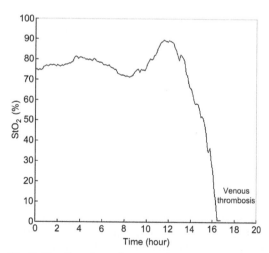

Fig. 9. The first sign of venous thrombosis picked up by the nursing staff was a drop in the tissue O_2 saturation. (*From* Keller A. Non-invasive tissue oximetry for flap monitoring: an initial study. J Reconstr Microsurg 2007;23:196; with permission.)

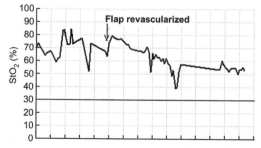

Fig. 8. The flap was revascularized at the arrow, but the StO_2 trended down. This tracing represents an early arterial thrombosis.

the sensor so that it does not move. The sensor can be secured either with the supplied adhesive backing, suturing it in place or with a transparent adhesive dressing. Carefully securing the sensor is important as it helps ensure that it will not move during the postoperative monitoring period. If the sensor moves, the continuity of the StO_2 trend data recorded on the monitor is interrupted and must be reestablished for a new representative spot on the flap. Signal quality assures consistency and reliability of readings during the postoperative monitoring period. If signal quality drops because of an event, such as dislodgement of the sensor, the monitor's alarm will sound and alert the clinician.

For 36 hours following the procedure the flap is continuously monitored. During that time patients will be out of bed, sitting in a chair, and able to ambulate around the bed. The sensor is removed after 36 hours to enable greater ease of ambulation.

MONITORING EXAMPLES

Sometimes movement of the flap can change the position of the vessels and cause them to kink and perhaps cause thrombosis. In this patient, the stretcher was placed in an upright position to transport the patient from the postoperative care

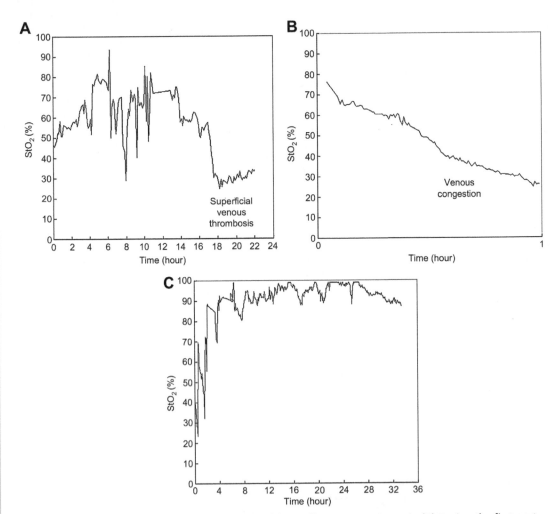

Fig. 10. This patient had thrombosis of the superficial (second) venous anastomosis. (A) During the first postoperative day, the tissue O_2 saturation fell. This decrease in the tissue O_2 saturation began before the flap took on a more congested appearance. (B) After revising the thrombosed venous anastomosis and returning to the recovery room, the tissue O_2 saturation rapidly fell without any change in flap appearance. The patient was returned to the operating room where the venous anastomosis was found to be thrombosed. It was again revised. (C) After the second revision of the venous anastomosis, the tissue O_2 saturation remained elevated above the pretransfer level for the next 36 hours. (*From* Keller A. Non-invasive tissue oximetry for flap monitoring: an initial study. J Reconstr Microsurg 2007;23:195; with permission.)

unit to the nursing floor. The vessels thrombosed while the patient was in an upright position (**Fig. 9**).

On some occasions there is not adequate venous drainage through the deep system and additional drainage through the superficial system becomes necessary. In this example, the superficial vein clotted while the patient was being monitored in the postoperative care unit. The StO_2 fell but not to a critical level. It was not until the flap showed signs of congestion, which included a bluish tinge, that the patient was re-explored. The venous anastomosis was revised and the patient was taken from the operating room with an elevated StO_2. Color of the flap also returned to normal. When the StO_2 again began to fall the patient was taken back to the operating room despite the fact that there were no new clinical findings. The superficial vein was again found to be thrombosed. The anastomosis was revised a second time. The flap and vessels were better positioned to maintain a patent superficial vein and the StO_2 returned to the preoperative values (**Fig. 10**). The patient had an uneventful recovery from this point without any evidence of fat necrosis.

Another patient who was undergoing postoperative monitoring went into a supraventricular tachycardia that did not respond to the usual intravenous medication. She deteriorated and eventually required cardiopulmonary resuscitation (CPR) and cardioversion. During the event there was an abrupt fall in the StO_2, which returned to normal when the patient went back into normal sinus rhythm (**Fig. 11**).

This example is of a patient who had a nonbreast free flap that was being monitored. The patient became agitated and clinical evaluation was performed. There were no specific findings and readings on the pulse oximeter were reported as normal. Retrospective examination of the StO_2 tracing showed that the oxygen saturation to the flap was slowly decreasing. Shortly thereafter, this patient had a respiratory and then cardiac arrest. With resuscitation, the flap StO_2 readings returned to normal (**Fig. 12**).

A hallmark of venous thrombosis is hematoma. Even without other clinical signs, the assumption is made that the vein draining the flap is clotted and the flap is decompressing itself. In this example, the patient had a large hematoma surrounding the flap but no change in the StO_2. Although this patient required an urgent return to the operating room to evacuate the hematoma and control the bleeding, there was a level of confidence based upon the lack of decline in the tissue oxygen saturation that the vascular anastomoses were intact and functioning (**Fig. 13**).

The author has previously reported in a study of 208 monitored flaps that with a fall of the StO_2 to less than 30% and a drop rate of greater than 20% in less than 30 minutes, a diagnosis of the occlusive event could be made within 1 hour of its onset.[14] In another study by Repez and colleagues,[2] 50 autologous tissue breast reconstructions were monitored continuously for 72 hours. Twenty percent of the flaps developed anastomotic thrombosis, which were identified using near infrared spectroscopy

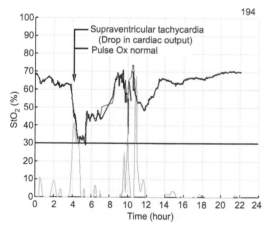

Fig. 11. A drop in StO_2 was measured in a patient experiencing supraventricular tachycardia in which cardiac output was reduced. (*From* Keller A. A new diagnostic algorithm for early prediction of vascular compromise in 208 microsurgical flaps using tissue oxygen saturation measurements. Ann Plast Surg 2009;62(5):542; with permission.)

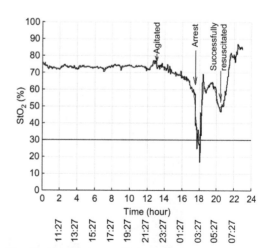

Fig. 12. This patient suffered a respiratory and then a cardiac arrest. He was successfully resuscitated. At point where he started to become agitated is noted. Note that his StO_2 shows a slight decline. He arrests and the StO_2 decreases dramatically He is successfully resuscitated and the StO_2 returns to pre-event values.

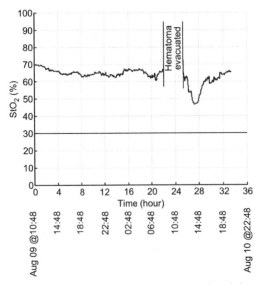

Fig. 13. This patient had a large hematoma that did not compromise flap perfusion. After the hematoma was evacuated, tissue oxygen saturation dropped slightly, which may have been physiologic or perhaps caused by flap manipulation, and then returned to the presurgical levels. This patient had an uneventful recovery.

monitoring. In all of these cases, the diagnosis was made using information from monitor and before it was clinically apparent.

ADDITIONAL USES OF TISSUE OXIMETRY IN FLAP ELEVATION

With increased confidence in the use of near infrared spectroscopy for the measurement of tissue oximetry additional uses of the technology have been explored. The determination of viability of portions of a flap is often problematic. Although plastic surgeons tend to make this decision based on the color of the tissue, the color and quality of the bleeding, and so forth, this is purely subjective. The use of near infrared tissue oximetry can aid in this decision-making process. The question routinely addressed is how much of zone 3 could be included in a flap based on the deep inferior epigastric system. The tissue oximetry sensor can be placed on different areas that are in question and StO$_2$ readings obtained. Areas with falling StO$_2$ levels are poorly perfused and cannot be included in the flap without increased risk of fat necrosis (**Fig. 14**).

Many patients who choose DIEP flap breast reconstruction have 1 or more abdominal scars. The issue of tissue viability distal to the scar can be answered in a similar fashion with the tissue oximeter. Sequential readings taken over time showed a drop in the StO$_2$ in certain areas of the flap and aid in making the determination of how much tissue to discard (**Fig. 15**).

Tissue oximetry may also be used in determining the need for an additional perforator to perfuse a flap. Before including or excluding that perforator, StO$_2$ measurements are obtained in different areas of the flap. The perforator in question is then occluded with a temporary clip and additional measurements are obtained. If there is no change in the StO$_2$ then that perforator may be divided and not included with the flap.

EVALUATION OF SKIN FLAPS

In immediate reconstruction, especially when a skin-sparing mastectomy has been done, viability

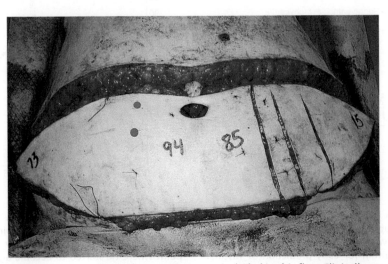

Fig. 14. The 2 green dots represent the perforators that were included in this flap. Clinically one would evaluate zones 3 and 4 based upon color and bleeding. The tissue oximeter was used to evaluate the different areas of the flap just before transfer.

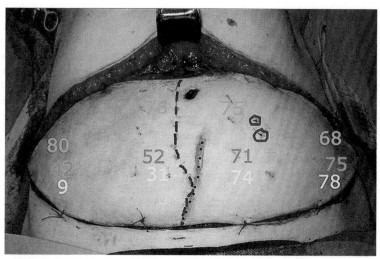

Fig. 15. The two included perforators are circled in red. The abdominal scar is marked with the dotted line. Sequential tissue oximetry readings were taken just after the flap was elevated, shown in green, 20 minutes after the flap was elevated, shown in blue, and 40 minutes after the flap was elevated, shown in yellow. The flap was divided along the dashed line. Note that even though the flap had good color just distal to the area where it was to be divided, the StO_2 readings had fallen significantly.

of the mastectomy skin flap must be determined. The clinical evaluation of color and bleeding sometimes does not provide enough information to reliably make this decision. This finding is especially true in darkly pigmented individuals or in bruised mastectomy flaps. Although it is always easy to excise more of the mastectomy skin, this often leads to a less satisfactory aesthetic result. In situations where the viability of the mastectomy skin is in question, StO_2 readings can be obtained from different areas along the mastectomy flaps. One will find a sharp demarcation marking where the healthy skin ends. This method has been used reliably in determining what mastectomy skin must be trimmed (**Fig. 16**).

SUMMARY

There is a clear trend today toward monitoring free flaps with new technology. Near infrared spectroscopy allows for a more rapid determination of vascular compromise than clinical evaluation. The use of tissue oximetry can aid in the determination of perforator selection and the amount of tissue that will survive on a given blood supply. Near infrared spectroscopy has also been useful in the evaluation of perfusion of mastectomy skin flaps.

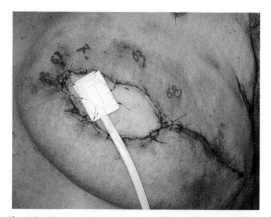

Fig. 16. Tissue oximetry was used to mark the mastectomy skin and identify areas that were not likely to survive. The skin was then trimmed using these numbers as a guide. Even though some skin appeared bruised, it had high StO_2 readings and was not trimmed. All of the mastectomy skin survived postoperatively.

REFERENCES

1. Keller A. A new diagnostic algorithm for early prediction of vascular compromise in 208 microsurgical flaps using tissue oxygen saturation measurements. Ann Plast Surg 2009;62(5):538–43.
2. Repez A, Oroszy D, Arnez ZM. Continuous postoperative monitoring of cutaneous free flaps using near infrared spectroscopy. J Plast Reconstr Aesthet Surg 2008;61:71–7.
3. Keller A. Perfusion zones of the DIEP flap revisited: a clinical study. Plast Reconstr Surg 2006;118(4):1076–7.
4. Siemionow M, Arslan E. Ischemia/reperfusion injury: a review in relation to free tissue transfers. Microsurgery 2004;24:468–75.

5. Jones NF. Intraoperative and postoperative monitoring of microsurgical free tissue transfers. Clin Plast Surg 1992;19:783–97.

6. Swartz WM, Izquierdo R, Miller MJ. Implantable venous Doppler microvascular monitoring: laboratory investigation and clinical results. Plast Reconstr Surg 1994;93:152–63.

7. Swartz WM, Jones NF, Cherup L, et al. Direct monitoring of microvascular anastomoses with the 20 MHz ultrasonic Doppler probe: an experimental and clinical study. Plast Reconstr Surg 1988;81:149–58.

8. Pestana IA, Coan B, Erdmann D, et al. Early experience with fluorescent angiography in free-tissue transfer reconstruction. Plast Reconstr Surg 2009; 123(4):1239–44.

9. Colwell A, Wright L, Karanas Y. Near-infrared spectroscopy measures tissue oxygenation in free flaps for breast reconstruction. Plast Reconstr Surg 2008;121(5):344e–5e.

10. Khouri RK. Avoiding free flap failure. Clin Plast Surg 1992;19:773–81.

11. Hirigoyen MB, Urken ML, Weinberg H, et al. Free flap monitoring: a review of current practice. Microsurgery 1995;16:723–7.

12. Smit JM, Zeebregts CJ, Acosta R, et al. Advancements in free flap monitoring in the last decade: a critical review. Plast Reconstr Surg 2010;125(1):177–85.

13. Hidalgo DA, Jones CS. The role of emergent exploration in free tissue transfer: a review of 150 consecutive cases. Plast Reconstr Surg 1990;89:492–8.

14. Keller A. Non-invasive tissue oximetry for flap monitoring: an initial study. J Reconstr Microsurg 2007; 23:189–98.

15. Thorniley MS, Sinclair JS, Barnett NJ, et al. The use of near-infrared spectroscopy for assessing the viability during reconstructive surgery. Br J Plast Surg 1998;51:218–26.

16. Mao JM, Wright L, Elmandjra M. Application of near infrared spectroscopy in monitoring blood perfusion in digital replantation. Proc SPIE 2005;5692:382–9.

17. Gimbel M, Rollins M, Fukaya E, et al. Monitoring partial and full venous outflow compromise in a rabbit skin model. Plast Reconstr Surg 2009; 124(3):796–803.

18. Najefi A, Leff DR, Nicolaou M, et al. Monitoring of free flaps using near-infrared spectroscopy: a systematic review of the initial trials. Plast Reconstr Surg 2010;125(4):182e–4e.

Index

Note: Page numbers of article titles are in **boldface** type.

A

Abdominal flap design, vascular information provided by magnetic resonance angiography for, 266–268
Abdominal wall flaps, anterior, 230–232
Anastomosis, microscopic, evaluation of, fluorescent angiography for, 297
Angiography, computed tomographic. See *Computed tomographic angiography.*
  fluorescent. See *Fluorescent angiography.*
  magnetic resonance. See *Magnetic resonance angiography.*

B

Breast reconstruction, autologous, acoustic Doppler sonography, color duplex ultrasound, and laser Doppler flowmetry for, **203–211**
  computed tomographic angiography and, 249
  flap monitoring in, 301
  maximizing use of handheld Doppler in, **213–218**
  near-infrared spectroscopy in, **301–307**
    background of, 301–302
  flaps and perforators used for, 265
  free tissue, use of implantable Doppler in, **309–312**
  perforator flap surgery in, 229
    recipient vessels for, 236–237
Buttock flaps, magnetic resonance angiography in use of, 268–270, 271, 272

C

Color-coded infrared thermograms, 277–278
Color Doppler imaging, 254
Color duplex ultrasound, 204, 206, 209
  acoustic Doppler sonography, and laser Doppler flowmetry, for autologous breast reconstruction, **203–211**
  basic physics of, 207
  for flap surgery, 167
Computed tomographic angiography, 213, 263
  and autologous breast reconstruction, 249
  and magnetic resonance angiography, for perforator-based free flaps, technical considerations in, **219–228**
  and multidetector row computed tomography, 243, 244, 246
    operative time, 246–247
  applications of, 219

  assessing outcomes of, **241–252**
  clinical applications of, **229–239**
  for preoperative imaging, 167–168
  future modalities of, 249
  image reconstruction from, 223–224
  multidetector row, 207–208, 209
  patient preparation for, 221–222
  performance of examination, 222
  technique of, 221, 230, 233
  volume rendered technique, 236, 237
Computed tomography, multidetector, 219
  multidetector row, 254
    and computed tomographic angiography, 243, 244, 246
    operative time, 246–247
Computed tomography scanning, dynamic (four-dimensional), 175–176
  static (three-dimensional), 176
Contrast-enhanced magnetic resonance angiography. See *Magnetic resonance angiography, contrast-enhanced.*

D

Donor site complications, related to perforator flaps, 235–236
Doppler, handheld, for flap reconstruction, postoperative monitoring following, 217
  in perforator selection, 215–216
  maximizing use of, in autologous breast resonstruction, **213–218**
  sequential clamping technique, 216–217
  standard unit, 214
  implantable, flap slavage rate, 310
  indications and settings for, 309–310
  reliability and value of, 310–311
  sensitivity of, 310–311
  specificity of, 311
  technique of, 309
  use in free tissue breast reconstruction, **309–311**
  preoperative transitioning, to intraoperative, 214–215
Doppler effect, 203
Doppler flowmetry, laser, 301
Doppler imaging, color, 254
Doppler physics, 214
Doppler sonography, acoustic, 203–204, 205, 209
  advantages of, 213
  basic physics of, 207

Clin Plastic Surg 38 (2011) 325–328
doi:10.1016/S0094-1298(11)00035-6
0094-1298/11/$ – see front matter © 2011 Elsevier Inc. All rights reserved.

Doppler (*continued*)
    color duplex ultrasound, and laser Doppler
        flowmetry, for autologous breast
        resonstruction, **203–211**
Doppler ultrasonography, 243–245
    in free-flap planning, 220
Duplex ultrasonography, 245–246
Dynamic infrared thermography, for vascular
    imaging, 169–170

E

Epigastric artery, deep inferior, perforator of, 230, 231
Epigastric artery flap, superficial inferior,
    230–232, 241

F

Flap circulation, postoperative assessment of, 171
Flap monitoring, tissue oximetry and, 319–320
Flap perfusion technologies, and perforator imaging,
    overview of, **165–174**
Flap surgery, duplex and color duplex
    ultrasonographies for, 167
    preoperative assessment for, 166–170
Flaps, and perforators, used for breast
    resonstruction, 265
    elevation of, tissue oximetry in, 322
Fluorescent angiography, 213, **293–295**
    applications of, 294–298
    for mapping of perforators, 170–171
    for postoperative monitoring, 297
    future directions in, 298
    in literature, 298
    technique of, 294
Fluorescent laser angiography, during perforator flap
    surgery, 294
Free flaps, perforator-based, comparison of
    techniques for, 225–226
        donor sites for, 230–234
        planning of, Doppler ultrasound in, 220

G

Gadolinium-containing contrast agents, 264
Gluteal artery perforator flap(s), 232
    superior and inferior, 194–197, 198
        anatomy of, 197, 198

I

Indocyanine green dye, 322–323
    advantages of, 322–323
Infrared thermography, dynamic, **277–292**
        history of, 277–278
        in intraoperative phase of deep inferior
            epigastric perforator flaps, 281–285,
            286, 287
        in preoperative phase of deep inferior
            epigastric perforator flaps, 279–281,
            282, 283
        postoperative use of, in deep inferior epigastric
            perforator flaps, 285–290
        use in reconstruction with free deep inferior
            epigastric perforator flap, 278–290
Intercostal artery perforator flap(s), 199, 200, 235–236
Interperforator flow, 176, 177

L

Laser Doppler flowmetry, 205–207, 208–209
Locoregional flap donor sites, 234–236
Lumbar artery perforator flap(s), 199–200

M

Magnetic resonance angiography, 213
    and computed tomographic angiography, for
        perforator-based free flaps, technical
        considerations in, **219–228**
    contrast-enhanced, **263–275**
        methods of, 264–265
        patients receiving, 265
        results of, 265–266
    current protocol for, 271–273
    finer points of, and perforator selection, 266–271
    for vascular imaging, 168–169
    image reconstruction from, 225, 226
    in use of buttock flaps, 270–271, 273
    in use of medial upper thigh flap, 270–271, 273
    patient positioning in scanner, 223
    patient preparation for, 222–223
    pulse sequences for, 223
    technique of, 222
    vascular information provided for, abdominal flap
        design by, 266–268
Magnetic resonance imaging, for preoperative
    perforator mapping, **253–261**
        discussion of, 258–260
        noncontrast, 254–258
Mammary artery, internal, perforator flaps, 234, 235
Medical documentation, protective, fluorescent
    angiography for, 297–298

N

Near-infrared spectroscopy, clinical applications
    of, 302–304
    for flap monitoring, 171, 172
    in autologous breast reconstruction, **301–307**
        background of, 301–302
        measurements by, 302
        intraoperative and postoperative monitoring
            of, 303, 304
        limitations of, 304–306
        tissue oximetry using, 313–314

O

Oximetry, tissue. See *Tissue oximetry*.

P

Perforasome(s), classification of, deep inferior
    epigastric perforator flaps and, 188–189, 193
    direct, and indirect linking vessels, 176
    theory of, 176–177
Perforating vessels, abdominal, preoperative study
    of, methods used for, 253–254
Perforator-based free flaps, computed tomographic
    angiography and magnetic resonance
    angiography for, technical considerations in,
    219–228
Perforator flap surgery, fluorescent laser angiography
    during, 294
    in breast reconstruction, 229
        recipient vessels for, 236–237
Perforator flap(s), 241–242
    complications related to, 247–248
    deep inferior epigastric, 166, 168, 230, 241
        anatomy of, 178
        and reappraisal of zones of perfusion, 183–186
        computed tomographic angiography for, 220
        dynamic infrared thermography in, in
            intraoperative phase, 281–285, 286, 287
            in preoperative phase, 279–281, 282, 283
            postoperative use of, 285–290
        harvest of, safe and unsafe zones of, 189
        lateral row, 182–183, 190, 191
            perforasome classification, 188–189, 193
        magnetic resonance angiography and, 220
        medial row, 178–180, 181–182
            perforasome classification, 188, 193
        single dominant medial row, 180–182, 184–189
        zones of perfusion, perforasome concept
            and, 187–188
    free deep inferior epigastric, dynamic infrared
        thermography with, 278–290
    gluteal artery, 232
        superior and inferior, 194–197, 198
            anatomy of, 197, 198
    intercostal artery, 199, 200, 235–236
    internal mammary artery, 234, 235
    lumbar artery, 199–200, 234
    selection of type and design of, 242–249
    thoracodorsal artery, 189–193, 195, 196
        anatomy of, 189
        disadvantages of, 189
    thoracostal artery, 236
Perforator imaging, and flap perfusion
    technology(ies), overview of, **165–174**
    and flap technology, 165–166
        historical overview of, 166
    intraoperative, 170–171

Perforator mapping, preoperative, magnetic
    resonance imaging for, **253–261**
        discussion of, 258–260
Perforator(s), and flaps, used for breast
    resonstruction, 265
    architecture of, assessing of, **175–202**
    deep inferior epigastric artery, 230, 231
    fluoresent angiography for mapping of, 170–171
    selection of, finer points of magnetic resonance
        angiography and, 266–271
Perfusion/angiosomes, tissue documenting of,
    fluorescent angiography for, 294–296
Perfusion flaps, and free-flap surgery, decision
    making in, fluorescent angiography for, 297
Preforator-based free flaps, comparison of
    techniques for, 225–226
    donor sites for, 230–234

R

Rectus abdominis myocutaneous flap(s), transverse,
    230, 242
        pedicled, 234–235

S

Skin flaps, evaluation of, 322–323
Spectroscopy, near-infrared, clinial applications of,
    302–304
        for flap monitoring, 171, 172
        in autologous breast reconstruction, **301–307**
            background of, 301–302
            measurements by, 302
            intraoperative and postoperative monitoring
                of, 303, 304
            limitations of, 304–306
            tissue oximetry using, 313–314
Superficial inferior epigastric artery flap, 230–232,
    241

T

Temperature, body, regulation of, 277, 278
Thermograms, infrared, color-coded, 277–278
Thermography, dynamic infrared. See *Infrared
    thermography, dynamic*.
Thigh flap, medial upper, magnetic resonance
    angiography in use of, 270–271, 273
Thoracodorsal artery perforator flap, 189–193,
    195, 196
        anatomy of, 189–193
        disadvantages of, 189
Thoracostal artery perforator flap, 236
Tissue oximeter, 314
Tissue oximetry, 315
    abnormal physiology, 315–319
    for flap monitoring, 319–320

Tissue oximetry (*continued*)
  in abnormal physiology, 315–319
  in flap elevation, 322
  in normal physiology, 315
  monitoring examples of, 320–322
  noninvasive, **313–324**
  using near-infrared spectroscopy, 313–314
Transverse rectus abdominis myocutaneous flap(s),
  230, 242
  pedicled, 234–235
Transverse upper gracilis flap, 232–234
  magnetic resonance angiography in use of,
    270–271, 273

U

Ultrasound, color duplex. See *Color duplex
  ultrasound*.
Upper gracilis flap, transverse, 232–234
  magnetic resonance angiography in use of,
    270–271, 273

V

Vascular anatomy, studying of, methods of, 175–176
Vascular system, deep inferior epigastric,
  computed tomographic angiography to
  study, 168

Moving?

Make sure your subscription moves with you!

To notify us of your new address, find your **Clinics Account Number** (located on your mailing label above your name), and contact customer service at:

Email: journalscustomerservice-usa@elsevier.com

800-654-2452 (subscribers in the U.S. & Canada)
314-447-8871 (subscribers outside of the U.S. & Canada)

Fax number: 314-447-8029

Elsevier Health Sciences Division
Subscription Customer Service
3251 Riverport Lane
Maryland Heights, MO 63043

*To ensure uninterrupted delivery of your subscription, please notify us at least 4 weeks in advance of move.

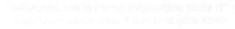

Printed and bound by CPI Group (UK) Ltd, Croydon, CR0 4YY

03/10/2024

01040357-0005